Experimental and Clinical Hepatology

Experimental and Clinical Hepatology

Proceedings of the 5th Workshop on
Experimental and Clinical Hepatology
held at Hannover, 23–24 November 1984

Edited by

Christof E. Brölsch

Department of Surgery
Section of Hepatobiliary Surgery
and Liver Transplantation
The University of Chicago, USA

and

Oskar Zelder

Zentrum für Operative Medizin I
Klinik für Allgemeinchirurgie
Philipps-Universität Marburg, West Germany

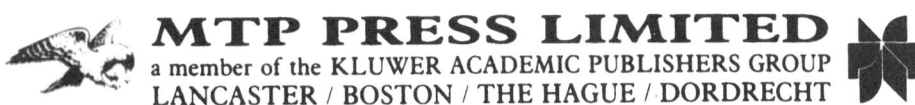

MTP PRESS LIMITED
a member of the KLUWER ACADEMIC PUBLISHERS GROUP
LANCASTER / BOSTON / THE HAGUE / DORDRECHT

Published in the UK and Europe by
MTP Press Limited
Falcon House
Lancaster, England

British Library Cataloguing in Publication Data

Workshop on Experimental and Clinical Hepatology
(5th : 1984 : Hannover)
Experimental and clinical hepatology : proceedings
of the 5th Workshop on Experimental and Clinical
Hepatology, Hannover, November 23,24 1984.
1. Liver—Diseases
I. Title   II. Brölsch, Christoph E.
III. Zelder, Oskar
616.3'62   RC845

ISBN-13: 978-94-010-8342-3   e-ISBN-13: 978-94-009-4151-9
DOI: 10.1007/978-94-009-4151-9

Published in the USA by
MTP Press
A division of Kluwer Boston Inc
190 Old Derby Street
Hingham, MA 02043, USA

Library of Congress Cataloging-in-Publication Data

Arbeitstagung Experimentelle und Klinische Hepatologie
(5th : 1984 : Hannover, Germany)
Experimental and clinical hepatology.

Summaries in German.
Includes bibliographies and index.
1. Liver—Diseases—Congresses.   2. Liver—Congresses.
I. Brölsch, Christoph E., 1944–   II. Zelder, Oskar.
III. Title. [DNLM: 1. Liver—congresses.   2. Liver
Diseases—congresses.   W3 AR135T 5th 1984e/WI 700 A664 1984e]
RC845.A68 1984   616.3'62   85–24096

Contents

v

SECTION 3   PORTAL CIRCULATION

SECTION 4   ISOLATED HEPATOCYTES

SECTION 5   LIVER PERFUSION

Preface

This is the fifth symposium on Experimental and Clinical Hepatology to be convened by the organisers, and, in common with the previous four, reflects the importance placed upon continuing discussion by clinical investigators as well as basic physiological and pharmacological researchers. Previous meetings which were held at the Surgical Department of the Philipps University in Marburg were dedicated to problems of direct clinical application, such as haemodynamics of portal hypertension, surgical approach to hepatic tumours, liver regeneration and temporary hepatic support. Clinical investigation was a subject which frequently came under discussion and some of these investigations have since lead to direct improvements in clinical therapy and many patients have benefited as a result.

This time, the convocation was called to the Medizinische Hochschule Hannover where remarkable advances in clinical liver transplantation have been the most striking event in clinical hepatology. The concensus of the meeting was that while significant clinical progress has been made, a variety of basic problems remained unsolved which will require further investigation. Special attention has, therefore, been given to topics such as acute liver damage, particularly within the transplanted liver, to chronic active hepatitis and its spontaneous prognosis, to isolated hepatocytes and their effect on functional support of the liver, to mechanisms of liver circulation which may be altered completely within the transplant and to liver perfusion which is still considered unsatisfactory for subsequent transplantation.

It was the aim of this conference to update and collect basic knowledge that can either be applied to further goals of liver transplantation or which requires special consideration and emphasis for future research. The papers presented at this meeting comprise this volume.

Sincere gratitude is expressed to the contributors who made the fifth symposium another success. The Editors are deeply indebted to Dr H. Noetzelmann, Merck A.G. and Dr H. Falk whose generous support made the meeting possible. We wish to thank Mr D. G. T. Bloomer, Managing Director of MTP Press Ltd for his superb cooperation in publishing these proceedings.

The Editors

List of Participants

ARMBRECHT, A., cand. med.
   Abt.für Nephrologie, Medizinische Hochschule Hannover
   Konstanty-Gutschow-Str. 8, D - 3000 Hannover

ASCHERL, R., Dr. med.
   Institut für Experimentelle Chirurgie, Technische
   Universität, Ismaninger Str. 22, D-8000 München

BALLE, C., Dr. med.
   Institut für Biochemie, Universität Göttingen
   Humboldtallee 23, D - 3400 Göttingen

BARTKOWSKI, R. Dr. med.
   Chirurgische Univ.-Klinik, Abteilung 2.1.1.,
   Im Neuenheimer Feld 110, D-6900 Heidelberg

BEUERS, U., Dr. med.
   Institut für Biochemie, Universität Göttingen
   Humboldtallee 23, D-3400 Göttingen

BÜTZOW, G., PD Dr. med.
   Med. Kern- und Poliklinik, Universitätskrankenhaus
   Eppendorf, Martinistr. 52, D-2000 Hamburg 20

BURGHARDT, M., cand. med.
   Abt. Gastroenterologie und Hepatologie,
   Medizinische Hochschule Hannover, D-3000 Hannover

BURGHOF, F., cand. med.
   Abt. Gastroenterologie und Hepatologie,
   Medizinische Hochschule Hannover, D-3000 Hannover

CHRIST, B., Dr. rer. nat.
   Institut für Biochemie, Universität Göttingen,
   Humboldtallee 23, D-3400 Göttingen

ENGEMANN, R., Dr. med.
    Abtl. für Allgemeinchirurgie,
    Christian-Albrechts Universität, D-2300 Kiel

GARDEMANN, A., Dr.rer. nat.
    Institut für Biochemie, Universität Göttingen
    Humboldtallee 23, D-3400 Göttingen

GRATZ, K., Dr. med.
    Abt. Gastroenterologie und Hepatologie,
    Medizinische Hochschule Hannover, D-3000 Hannover

HENNE-BRUNS, D., Dr. med.
    Chirurgische Klinik, Universitätskrankenhaus Eppendorf,
    Martinistr. 52, D-2000 Hamburg 20

JERUSALEM, C., Prof. Dr. med.
    Institut Zytologie und Histologie,
    Geert Grotteplein N 21, 6500 HB Nijmegen,Niederlande

KATZ, N., Dr. med.
    Zentrallabor am Klinikum, Universität Freiburg
    Hugstetter-Str. 55, D-7800 Freiburg

KIRN, A., Prof. Dr. med.
    Laboratoire de Virologie, Faculte Medicine,
    3, rue Koeberlé, 6700 Strasburg, Frankreich

KOUSSOURIS, P.,
    Department für Chirurgie und Gefäßchirurgie
    Heinz-Kalk-Klinik, D-8730 Bad Kissingen

LENG-PESCHLOW, E., Dr. med.
    c/o Madaus & Co., Abt. Pharmakologie, D-5000 Köln

LESER, H., Dr. med.
    Medizinische Universitätsklinik Freiburg
    Hugstetter-Str. 55, D-7800 Freiburg

LÖSGEN, H., Dr. med.
    Abt. Gastroenterologie und Hepatologie,
    Medizinische Hochschule Hannover, D-3000 Hannover

MEYER ZUM BÜSCHENFELDE, K.H., Prof. Dr. Dr.
    Leiter der I.Medizinischen Klinik und Poliklinik
    der Johannes-Gutenberg Universität Mainz,
    Langenbeckstr. 1, D-6500 Mainz

MÜLLER, G., Dr. med.
    Chirurgische Universität Tübingen
    Calwer Str. 7, D-7400 Tübingen

MÜTING, Dr., Prof. Dr. med.
    Dept.Innere Medizin und Gastroenterologie,
    Heinz-Kalk-Klinik, D-8730 Bad Kissingen

OTTO, G., Doz.Dr.sc. med.
   Chirurgische Klinik der Charité
   1040 Berlin, DDR

PAQUET, K., Prof. Dr. med.
   Department für Chirurgie und Gefäßchirurgie,
   Heinz-Kalk-Klinik, D-8730 Bad Kissingen

SCHMIDT, E., Prof. Dr.med.
   Abt.Gastroenterologie und Hepatologie,
   Medizinische Hochschule Hannover, D-3000 Hannover

SCHNEIDER, M., Dr. med.
   Medizinische Univ.-Klinik, Abt. B
   Albert-Schweitzer-Str. 35, D-4400 Münster

SCHÖLMERICH, M., Dr. med.
   Medizinische Universitätsklinik, Hugstetter-Str.
   D-7800 Freiburg

SCHRAUT, H., M.D.
   University of Chicago, Department of Surgery,
   5841 S.Maryland Avenue, Chicago, Illinois 60637, USA

STARITZ, M., Dr. med.
   I. Medizinische Klinik und Poliklinik,
   Johannes-Gutenberg-Universität, D-6500 Mainz

STEFFEN, Ch., Dr. med.
   Institut für Pharmakologie und Toxikologie,
   Philipps-Universität Marburg, Lahnberge, D-3550 Marburg

VELASQUEZ, D., Dr. med.
   Abt. Gastroenterologie und Hepatologie,
   Medizinische Hochschule Hannover, D-3000 Hannover

WALTER, C., Dr. med.
   Klinikum Steglitz der FU Berlin,
   Abt. Allgemein-, Gefäß- und Thoraxchirurgie,
   D-1000 Berlin 45

WITTIG, B., Dr. rer. nat.
   Institut für Biochemie, Universität Göttingen,
   Humboldtallee 23, D-3400 Göttingen

WULFFEN, von, H., Dr. med.
   Institut für Mikrobiologie, UKE Hamburg,
   Martinistr. 52, D-2000 Hamburg 20

Liver Injury

Liver Injury

1
Changes of the Energy – Metabolism in Liver Tissue After Experimental Common Bile Duct Obstruction

R. ASCHERL, J. MÜLLER, G. METAK, C. HÖSS*, P. WENDT
and G. BLÜMEL

*Institut für Experimentelle Chirurgie und *Frauenklinik der Technischen Universität München*

Zusammenfassung

Nach experimentell induzierter Choledochusstenose wurden die Adeninnukleotide ATP, ADP und AMP sowie Laktat und Pyruvat im Lebergewebe gemessen. Nach zwei Tagen post operationem war der Gehalt an ATP auf 40 %, der 'energy charge' auf zwei Drittel sowie Pyruvat auf 60 % der Normalwerte gesunken, AMP auf das Vierfache der Normal- werte gestiegen. Bei sham-operierten Tieren fand sich wenige Stunden nach der Operation ein den ligierten Tieren entsprechendes Muster, nach zwei Tagen post opera- tionem zeigte sich eine Angleichung an die Normalwerte.

Objectives

Patients with obstructive jaundice have a high incidence of postoperative complications as well as mortality (3). The fragile homeostatic equilibrium of the hepatic metabolism is severely impaired by the extrahepatic bile duct obstruction.
The effects of extrahepatic biliary obstruction on the energy-metabolism of the liver were studied in rats in order to define some of the alterations in the liver metabolism (4).

Material and Methods

Healthy male Wistar rats (300 - 400 g BW) were divided
into seven groups: group 1 had no operation, for each
postoperative period (4, 24, and 48 h, resp.) we had one
group of operated and one group of sham-operated animals
(n = 6 to 8 per group). After a median laparotomy under
general anaesthesia with ketamine and xylacine the
proximal common bile duct was dissected and ligated
twice with 3-0 catgut. In the sham-groups we used non-
occluding loops of 3-0 catgut instead of ligatures. After
the defined postoperative periods the liver was clamped
and frozen in situ with special tongs precooled in liquid
nitrogen, powdered in a bath of liquid nitrogen and homo-
genized with perchloric acid. The content of adenine
nucleotides, lactate, and pyruvate was measured in the
supernatant (2). The 'energy charge' was calculated
according to the formula by ATKINSON (1):

$$\frac{ATP + 1/2\ ADP}{ATP + ADP + AMP}$$

Results

ATP :

After 4 h concentrations decreased significantly in both
groups. 24 and even more 48 h postoperatively levels in
operated animals decreased further to 40 % of normal
values, whereas levels in sham-operated animals
recovered to 85 % of normal values.

ADP :

No significant changes in either group.

AMP :

After 4 h concentrations increased in both groups. 24
and 48 h postoperatively levels of the sham-groups
decreased to almost normal values, whereas in operated
animals we found an increase to almost four times the
normal values.

'Energy charge' :

The 'energy charge' decreased slightly in both groups
after 4h. 48 h postoperatively it was reduced to 60 % of

normal values in ligated animals, whereas we found almost
normal levels in the sham-groups.

Lactate :

No significant changes in either group.

Pyruvate :

After 4 h concentrations were up to twice the normal
levels in both groups. 48 h postoperatively levels in
ligated animals decreased to 35 % of normal values,
whereas we found almost normal levels in the sham-groups.

Discussion

Our results indicate a massive metabolic disturbance in
the obstructed liver. To evaluate the viability of the
liver function after common bile duct obstruction, we used
the 'energy charge' proposed by ATKINSON (1) as a parameter, because the metabolic functions of the liver depend
on the continuous supply of energy, i.e. ATP. The 'energy
charge' is of central importance in correlating metabolic
functions and maintaining metabolic stability necessary
for life (2, 4). In this dynamic steady state, a rise in
the energy expenditure of the cells would result in a
decrease of the 'energy charge' unless it is accompanied
by a concomitant increase in the rate of phosphorylation
of AMP/ADP to ATP. In a state of high energy demand more
ATP is produced by glycolysis via pyruvate avoiding the
energy-demanding pathway via lactate.
The marked decrease in the energy charge of the obstructed
liver indicates, that a metabolic overload demanding
energy is being imposed upon the liver. After 1 and 2 days
the gradual pressure increase in the prestenotic biliary
tract and the intracellular increase of substances usually
excreted into the bile impose a metabolic burden on the
obstructed liver. As most bile components are transported
actively the liver cells have to excrete the bile
components against a higher concentration gradient and
therefore need more energy. The oxidative phosphorylation
might be impaired by the rising concentration of cell-toxic

Table: Adenine-nucleotides, 'energy charge', and pyruvate in the liver tissue of rats after extrahepatic biliary obstruction

		ATP (μmol/ml)	AMP (μmol/ml)	'energy charge'	pyruvate (μmol/ml)
no operation	n=11	3.70 + 0.52	0.36 + 0.09	0.79 + 0.04	0.13 + 0.06
4 h after ligation	n=6	2.13 + 0.62	0.52 + 0.13	0.67 + 0.05	0.30 + 0.11
4 h after sham	n=6	2.68 + 0.37	0.65 + 0.17	0.67 + 0.01	0.23 + 0.15
24 h after ligation	n=7	2.03 + 0.57**	1.49 + 0.27**	0.52 + 0.06**	0.20 + 0.05
24 h after sham	n=8	3.11 + 0.82	0.65 + 0.20	0.68 + 0.06	0.15 + 0.03
48 h after ligation	n=7	1.44 + 0.38**	1.28 + 0.18**	0.51 + 0.05**	0.08 + 0.02*
48 h after sham	n=7	3.10 + 0.22	0.38 + 0.08	0.73 + 0.02	0.14 + 0.06

* $p \leq 0.05$;   ** $p \leq 0.01$;   mean values ± SD

bile components and therefore be a further reason for the decrease of ATP and the 'energy charge'.

References

1. Atkinson, D.E. (1968): The energy charge of the adenylate pool as a regulatory parameter, interaction with feed back modifiers. Biochemistry, 7: 4030 - 4038

2. Bergmeyer, H.U. (1970): Methoden der enzymatischen Analyse. Verlag Chemie Weinheim, p. 1491-1496, 1510-1514, 2020-2033, 2178-2181

3. Dunphy, J.E., Way, L.W. (1981): Biliary tract. In: Current Diagnosis & Treatment, ed.: Dunphy, J.E. and Way, L.W., Lange Medical Publications, p.475-503

4. Ozawa, K. et al. (1979): Early metabolic or common bile duct obstruction in rabbits. Eur. Surg. Res.,11, 61 - 70

Reprints to :

Dr. med. Rudolf Ascherl
Institut für Experimentelle Chirurgie der TU-München
Ismaninger Str. 22
D - 8000 München 80
F.R.G.

2
Enzymatic Detoxification of Endogenous Toxins *In Vitro* and *In Vivo*

D. VELASQUEZ, K. BELSNER and G. BRUNNER

Abtl. für Gastroenterologie und Hepatologie, Medizinische Hochschule Hannover

Zusammenfassung

Mit der neuen lipophilen Hohlfasertechnik wurden die endogenen Toxine Phenol, Paracresol und Dodecansäure enzymatisch entgiftet. Toxinhaltiges Blut oder Serum wird durch die lipophilen Hohlfasern gepumpt. Eine Kofaktor enthaltende Enzymlösung circuliert auf der anderen Seite der lipophilen Hohlfasermembran. Die lipophilen Toxine akubolieren innen und wandern durch die Lipidmembran. Durch enzymatische Hydroxilierung oder Konjugation werden die lipophilen Toxine in eine hydrophile Substanz umgewandelt und können so nicht mehr in das Blut zurückdefundieren. Die von den Aminosäuren Thyrosin, Tryptophan und Phenylanin herrührenden Toxine Phenol und Paracresol wurden in vitro mit der UDP-Glucuronyltransferase und der Sulfattransferase entgiftet. Zur in vivo-Entgiftung des Phenol wurde die UDP-Glucuronyltransferase verwendet. Die transmembranösen Glucuronidierungsraten betrugen für Phenol und Paracresol 30 und 55 pmol/mg protein/h/cm^2 Hohlfaserfläche. Die Sulfatierung von Phenol und Cresol mit der Sulfattransferase betrug 38 und 47 pmol/mg protein/h/cm^2.
Die toxische Fettsäure Dodecansäure wurde in vitro mit dem Cytochrom-P-450 und der Cytochrom-P-450-Reduktase

hydroxiliert. Die transmembranöse Hydroxilierungsrate
betrug 625 pmol/h/nmol cytochrom-P-450/cm^2.
Mit dieser Technik können endogene Toxine unspezifisch
enzymatisch aus dem Blut entfernt werden, ohne daß
Immunreaktionen durch das Enzymprotein ausgelöst werden.
Die Toxine können frei zum Enzym hin defundieren,
während das Blut vom Enzym durch die Membran getrennt
bleibt.

Materials and methods

0,3 mM toxin solutions were prepared by adding phenol,
p-cresol and dodecanoids acid to human serum.
For the in vivo experiments a buffered 0,3M solution was
pumped into the ear vein of a male rabbit at a rate of
0,014 mmole/min/kg bodyeight. When the animal went into
coma after approximately 20 minutes the infusion rate was
reduced to 0,037 mmole/min/kg in order to maintain a
steady coma state.
UDP-glucuronyltransferase was prepared in crude form from
pig liver microsomes as previously described (1). For
sulfate reactions rabbit liver cytosole was prepared by
standard techniques.
Lipid hollow fiber modules with a membrane surface of
76 cm^2 were purchased from Fresenius AG (Bad Homburg/
Germany).
Toxin solutions were pumped through the hollow fiber at
rates of 8 ml/minute. The enzyme solutions were pumped
at rates of 10,5 ml/minute.
The measurements of phenyl glucuronide and cresol
glucuronide were carried out by isotachophoresis as
previously described (2). Dodecanoid acid and OH-
dodecanoic acid and OH-dodecanoic acid were measured by
HPLC as follows:
After derivatisation of the ether extracts with
phenacetylbromide in acetonitrile (56°C, 2 hours;
katalyst tributylamine) the samples were subjected to
HPLC. (Solvent system A: 50 % methanol in H$_2$O; solvent

system B: 100 % methanol) Separation was achieved by a
gradient of 60 % - 90 % solvent B within 10 minutes
followed by isocratic elution with 90 %. B. Bolumn:
Nucleosil 5C18, 250 mm, ∅ 4 mm, flow rate 1 ml/min;
UV detection at 260 nm.

For in vivo studies the access to the vascular system of
male rabbits was performed at the femoral artery and vein.
The natural force of the arterial flow was sufficient to
drive the blood through the hollow fiber device. It was
pumped back to the animal from the collection vessel
(Fig. 1) by a roller pump.

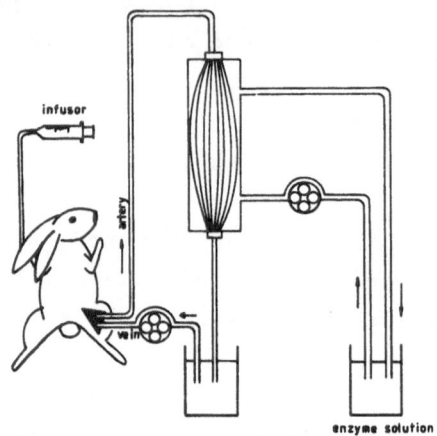

Fig. 1:   Experimental setup of phenol intoxication and
           enzymatic glucuronidation in a male rabbit.
           For details see "materials and methods"

Phenol and p-cresol were determined by gas chromato-
graphie:

To 0.9 ml sample (serum or buffer solution) 0.1 ml 25 mM
dinitrophenol was added as internal standard. 3.0 ml
ethanol and 0.15 ml 1n H_2SO_4 were added and the mixture
was shaken for 10 min and then zentrifuged at 5000 rpm
for 10 min.

To 3.0 ml supernatant 1.5 ml 10 % H_3PO_4 was added and the
mixture stirred for 10 min and then zentrifuged at
5000 rpm for 10 min.

To 1.5 ml supernatant 1.5 ml distilled water and 6.0 ml
CCL_4 were added an mixed for 30 minutes. After settling
5 ul of the organic phase was injected into a gas
chromatograph model Packard 438. Detector PID-HNM, lamp
temperature $220^{\circ}C$, carrier flow N_2 15 ml/min. Injection
temp. $200^{\circ}C$. Detector temp. $225^{\circ}C$, oven temp. $150^{\circ}C$,
Column 2.5 m, 2mm inner diameter filled with 3 % Hi-Eff-
8BP on Gas-Chrom Q 125-150 mesh.

Results

In figure 2a a typical in vitro experiment is shown.
Phenol concentration decreases with time on the toxin
side, while phenylglucuronide increases in concentration
on the enzyme side. Figure 2b shows a typical in vivo
experiment. While the blood level of phenol cannot be
judged because of the continous infusion of phenol.

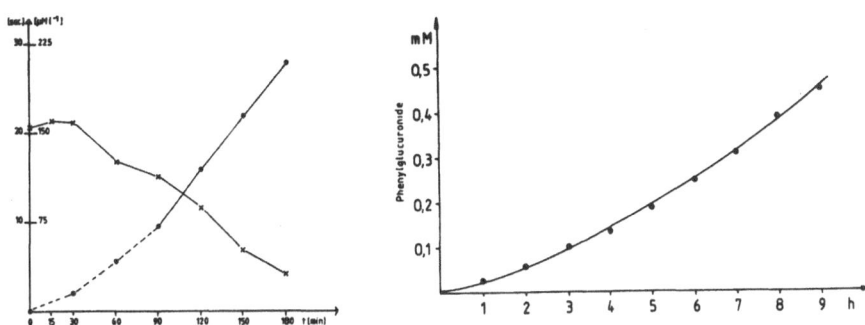

Fig. 2$_{a+b}$: (a) In vitro glucuronidation of phenol
containing serum in a lipophilic hollow fiber
experiment. Decrease of phenol concentration
on the toxins side is followed by an increase
of phenylglucuronide on the enzyme side.
(b) Formation of phenylglucuronide on the
enzyme side in the experiment shown in
figure 1.

The steady increase of phenylglucuronide formed can be
seen on the enzyme side. The transmembranous catalytic
rates for the different enzymes and toxins tested are
listed on table 1.

Table 1: Transmembranous catalytic rates for the
         enzymatic detoxification of some endogenous
         toxins occuring in liver failure

Enzyme	Toxin	pmol/mg/h/cm^2 membrane surface
UDP-glucuronyl-	Phenol	30
transferase	p-cresol	55
Sulfatetransferase	Phenol	38
	p-cresol	47
Cytochrome-p-450	Dodecanoic acid	625 (pmol/h/nmol p-450/cm^2)

The transmembranous glucuronidation with different
membrane surface and different membrane thickness is
demonstrated in figure 3.

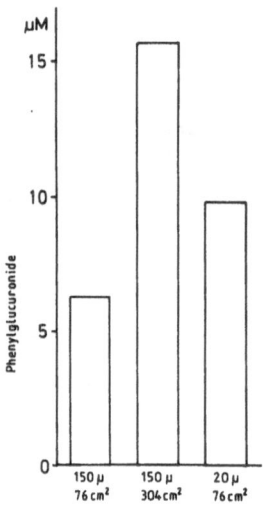

Fig. 3: Transmembranous production of phenylglucuronide
        in relation to membrane surface and membrane
        thickness. μmol phenylglucuronide formed during
        a 5 hour experiment. Phenol concentration =
        0,3 mmol/l circulated at 3,5 ml/min. Cofactor-
        enzyme solution circulated at 0,9 ml/min.

The amount of toxin removed increases with increasing membrane surface. This increase is however not directly proportional to the increase in membrane surface. The same applies to a decrease in membrane thickness.

Discussion

The experiments show that with the lipid hollow fiber technique toxins can be specifically removed from blood in vitro and in vivo by enzymes without immunological hazzards.

The transmembranous enzymatic detoxification is limited by the transmembranous transfer of toxins which can be demonstrated by the increase in detoxification rate when the membrane surface is increased or the membrane thickness is decreased. From the transmembranous catalytic rate shown in table 1 it can be calculated that 4 hours of hollow-fiber-enzyme treatment are needed to clear the serum (3 liters) of a patient from a 0,3 mM phenol concentration when $1m^2$ fiber surface and 100 ml enzyme solution with a protein content of 10 mg/ml are used. Since similar phenol concentrations are observed in severe hepatic disease it seems feasable that such treatment could be used as a support in liver failure. Large amounts of lipophilic toxins are "hidden" in fat tissue and cell membranes. These are in equilibrium with their serum levels and rediffuse or reenter the serum of the patients when the serum levels are lowered by hollow fiber enzyme treatment. Therefore treatment would have to be longer than could be calculated from the serum concentrations of the toxins. The experiments have to be extended for more groups of toxins and their corresponding enzymes and it is still a long way before enzymes can be used efficiently for the removal of toxins in liver failure.

References

1. Brunner, G., Holloway, C.J. and Lösgen, H. (1979).
   Large agarose beads for extracorporeal detoxification
   systems. 2. Preparation and enzymatic properties of
   agarose-bound UDP-glucuronyltransferase.
   Int. J. Artif. Organs. 2, 163

2. Brunner, G. and Holloway, C.J. (1980).
   The Capillary-Isotachophoretic Analysis of Reactants
   and Products of Clucuronidation. A New Method for the
   Assay of UDP-glucuronosyltransferase.
   Hoppe-Seyler's Z.Physiol. Chem. Bd. 381, 1

Reprints to :

Prof.Dr.med.G.Brunner
Abt. Gastroenterologie und Hepatologie
Medizinische Hochschule Hannover
D - 3000 Hannover

3

On the Position of the Determination of Bile Acids in Serum (Fasting = FBA and After a Standardized Test Meal = PPBA) in the Laboratory Diagnosis of Liver Diseases

F. BURGHOF, A. KELBER, J. LOBERS, E. SCHMIDT and F.W. SCHMIDT

Abt. Gastroenterologie und Hepatologie, Zentrum Innere Medizin und Dermatologie, Medizinische Hochschule, Hannover, F.R.G.

Zusammenfassung

1. Bei 151 Patienten mit Leber- und Gallenwegs-Erkrankungen wurde die diagnostische Aussage der Serum-Gallensäuren-Konzentration (nüchtern und nach standardisierter Test-Mahlzeit) mit der eines Standard-Enzym-Profils im Serum verglichen.

2. Bei akuter Virushepatitis, Verschluss-Ikterus und Lebercirrhose war die diagnostische Sensitivität der Gallensäuren der des Enzym-Profils vergleichbar, bei leichten Leberschäden, chronischer Hepatitis und Leber-Tumoren unterlegen.

3. Die diagnostische Sensitivität der postprandialen Gallensäuren-Konzentration war der Nüchtern-Gallensäuren-Konzentration bei der chronischen Hepatitis überlegen, bei Verschluss-Ikterus und Leber-Tumoren unterlegen.

4. Durch Gallensäuren-Bestimmungen zusätzlich zum Enzym-Profil kann mittels Diskriminanz-Analyse die korrekte Klassifikation von Einzelpatienten bei 4 von 9 differential-diagnostischen Fragestellungen verbessert werden.

Recently, the former enthusiasm for the determination of bile acids in Serum as the most sensitive and specific liver test (1, 2) has markedly abated (3, 4). In

parallel, the superiority of PPBA as compared to FBA has
also been challenged (5, 6).

We began a study with the aim to answer three questions:

1. Which liver disease can be detected better by the
determination of bile acids (BA) in serum than by the
standard enzyme profile?

2. Can the determination of bile acids improve the
differential diagnosis of liver diseases beyond the
informations given by the standard enzyme profile?

3. Has the determination of PPBA after a standarized test
meal a higher diagnostic sensitivity or specificity and
better predictive values than that of FBA?

Material and Methods

151 in- and outpatients of the MHH with diseases of the
liver and the biliary system were investigated. Their
classification is shown in Table 1. The FBA and PPBA
levels of the healthy controls were estimated by
H. POHLABELN (Diss. MHH 1985).

FBA and PPBA were determined enzymatically with 3-alpha-
hydroxy-steroid dehydrogenase (Enzabile[R], Nyegaard, Oslo
and Merck, Darmstadt).

CV within run: 3.6 %; CV between runs: 5.6 %.

Upper reference limits: FBA = 6 μmol/l; PPBA = 30 μmol/l.

The gallbladder empytying was induced by 20 gms of
Biloptin Reizmahlzeit[R] (Schering, Berlin) on the eve of
the test, and, on the following morning after taking
the blood sample for FBA with the double dose
(2 x 10 g dried egg's yolk + 2 x 8.95 g sorbitol).
The blood samples for PPBA were taken 2 hours
afterwards.

Table 1 :

PATIENTS	n	% pathological values								
		FBA	PPBA	ASAT	ALAT	GLDH	LDH	GGT	ALP	CHE
Acute viral hepatitis (ASAT and ALAT ►200 U/l)	14	100	100	100	100	100	100	93	93	50
Acute viral hepatitis (ASAT or ALAT ◄200 U/l)	9	89	89	100	100	100	44	100	89	44
Chronic persistent hepatitis	8	25	50	62	50	25	50	62	12	50
Chronic active hepatitis	6	33	67	83	83	67	33	67	50	0
Chronic active hepatitis with incipient cirrhosis	10	60	80	80	80	70	20	80	30	40
Hepatic and cryptogenetic cirrhosis	14	86	100	64	57	7	29	86	50	50
Alcoholic fatty liver	9	0	0	11	22	32	33	56	11	67
Chronic alcohol toxic hepatitis	7	14	14	71	71	43	57	100	14	43
Alcohol toxic cirrhosis	6	67	83	50	50	33	50	67	83	67
Cirrhosis with ascites (all types)	16	100	100	94	81	50	75	87	68	100
Primary biliary cirrhosis	11	91	91	100	100	100	45	100	100	45
Primary hepatoma	9	78	44	67	89	89	62	100	89	67
Liver metastases	11	18	20	36	27	64	80	64	45	54
Biliary obstruction	14	100	86	100	100	93	72	100	100	64
Chronic cholangitis	2	50	50	50	100	100	50	100	100	100
Morbus Gilbert	5	0	60	0	0	0	0	0	20+	0
CONTROLS (healthy adults, 20 – 76 years)	26	0	0	0	0	0	0	0	0	0

+ 1 young male, still growing (bone isoenzyme)

Results and Discussion

Fig. 1 shows how frequently FBA and PPBA concentrations
were elevated in the sera of all patients, as compared to
7 enzymes, which have been measured in parallel. The
diagnostic sensitivity of FBA is slightly less, that of
PPBA slightly more than 70 %, comparable to the aminotransferase, not reached by GLDH and ALP, let alone LDH
and CHE, but surpassed by GGT.

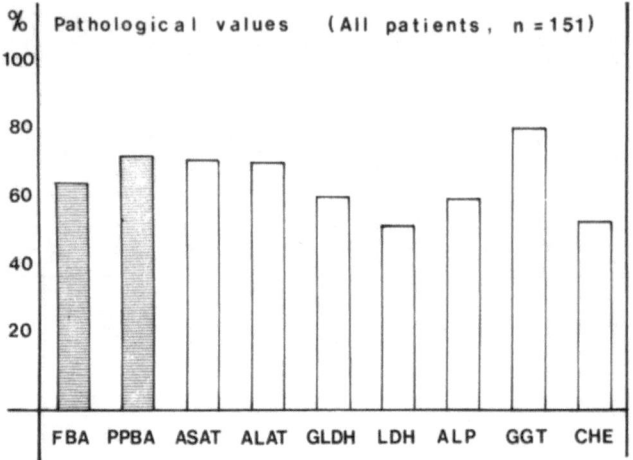

Fig. 1: Bile acid concentrations and enzyme activities in
        serum of 151 patients with diseases of the liver
        and the biliary system: Prevalence of patholo-
        gical values.
        FBA = fasting bile acids; PPBA = postprandial
        bile acids; ASAT = apsartate aminotransferase
        (E.C. 2.6.1.1); ALAT = alanine aminotransferase
        (E.C. 2.6.1.2); GLDH = glutamate dehydrogenase
        (E.C. 1.4.1.3); LDH = Lactate dehydrogenase
        (E.C. 1.1.1.27); ALP = alkaline phosphatase
        (E.C. 3.1.3.1); GGT = gamma-glutamyl transferase
        (E.C. 2.3.2.2); CHE = cholinesterase
        (E.C. 3.1.1.8).

An overall information of this kind is obviously of limited value. Therefore, in Table I the individual disease entities are listed separately. It can be seen that in chronic inflammations of the liver, viral or toxic in origin, in the earlier and milder stages, the diagnostic sensitivity of BA is clearly lower than that of enzyme activities in serum; whereas in the late stages, the cirrhoses and in primary carcinoma of the liver, the sensitivity of BA reaches or surpasses that of the amino-transferases or GGT.

In acute viral hepatitis the diagnostic sensitivity of BA determinations is as high as in cirrhosis. The intra- and extrahepatic obstructive cholestases, however, differ widely: from less than 20 % elevated levels of BA in metastatic liver disease up to more than 90 % in extra-hepatic obstruction. For the diagnosis of liver tumors and cholangitis enzyme determinations are clearly superior to BA estimations. Comparing the prevalence of pathological results of FBA and PPBA, there is sometimes no difference, e.g. in acute viral and chronic toxic hepatitis, or primary biliary and very advanced cirr-hosis, or cholangitis. In chronic persistent and chronic active hepatitis and in alcoholic cirrhosis, PPBA deter-mination detects up to twice as many patients than that of FBA. In contrast, in primary hepatoma and, less so, in extrahepatic obstruction, PPBA are less frequently in their pathological range than are FBA.

Table II shows the extent of PPBA elevations in serum in chronic inflammatory and in cholestatic liver diseases in multiples of their respective upper reference limits, and the ratios PPBA / FBA.

The relative rises of FBA and PPBA are similar and not marked in chronic hepatitis. They are more pronounced in cirrhosis of all types, and here, the elevations of FBA is twice that of PPBA, relatively. There is a rough correlation between prevalence and extent of alteration. This is also true for the cholestatic conditions, which

begin with primary biliary cirrhosis, belonging likewise
to the inflammatory diseases. The intrahepatic cholestases due to tumors, have relatively low increases of BA,
whereas extrahepatic obstruction shows the highest values
of FBA as well as PPBA. Nevertheless, the postprandial
increase is weaker than normal in all these conditions.

Table 2 :   Relative Elevations of FBA and PPBA in chronic
             inflammatory and cholestatic liver diseases
             and ratios of PPBA / FBA

	FBA: x normal	PPBA: x normal	PPBA/FBA (Mean)
Chronic alcoholic hepatitis	1.4 x	1.0 x	4.4
Chronic persistent hepatitis	4.8 x	4.5 x	5.4
Chronic active hepatitis	13 x	6.3 x	7.1
Alcohol toxic cirrhosis	22 x	15 x	4.0
Hepatitis cirrhosis	25 x	11 x	2.5
Cirrhosis with ascites	22 x	11 x	2.9
Primary biliary cirrhosis	23 x	10 x	2.6
Liver metastases	7 x	2.6 x	2.2
Primary hepatoma	12 x	4.2 x	2.1
Extrahepatic obstruction	54 x	13 x	1.4

As a rule, the significance of BA for the differential
diagnosis of liver diseases is considered negligible.
So, it came to us as a surprise that the addition of the
results of BA determinations to the standard enzyme
profile enhanced the accuracy of prediction in nearly
half of the differential diagnostic problems examined so
far.

Table III shows the results of the discriminant analysis
of 9 differential diagnostic problems, each with 4
possible diagnoses to choose from. The numbers to the
left refer to the correct classifications by the enzyme
pattern alone, the right ones indicate the improvement of
accuracy by addition of the bile acid concentrations in
serum.

Table 3 :   Improvement of differential diagnosis by
             enzyme patterns through addition of bile
             acid determinations

Correct classification by discriminant analysis

Differential diagnosis improved

Stages of chronic viral hepatitis	50 ➡ 67 %
Obstructive cholestasis	64 ➡ 81 %
Minimal liver lesions	55 ➡ 68 %
Early acute viral hepatitis	76 ➡ 84 %
Different types of cirrhosis	83 ➡ 86 %

Differential diagnosis not improved

Stages of chronic toxic hepatitis	76 = 76 %
Different types of chronic hepatitis	76 = 76 %
Subsiding acute viral hepatitis	78 = 78 %
Fatty liver	79 = 79 %

The best result was achieved for the staging of chronic viral hepatitis, only minimal or no improvement was found for the etiological classification.

Summary and conclusions

1. The diagnostic sensitivity of total bile acid determination is above 80 % and comparable to that of the
   standard enzyme profile in hepatology only in acute
   viral hepatitis, obstructive jaundice and liver
   cirrhosis.

2. It is inferior to that of standard enzyme determinations in slight liver lesions, liver tumors and
   chronic hepatitis.

3. In chronic hepatitis the diagnostic sensitivity of
   PPBA is clearly superior to the of FBA. In liver
   tumors and in obstructive jaundice the opposite is
   true.

4. Correct classification of individual patients by
   discriminant analysis can be improved significantly in
   4 out of 9 examined differential diagnostic settings
   by addition of bile acid determinations to the determination of the standard enzyme profile.

References

1. Carey, JB, Williams, G. (1963): J. Clin. Invest. 42, 450

2. Wildgrube, H.J., Stang, H., Winkler, M., Mauritz, G. (1982): Dtsch.med. Wschr. 107, 1235

3. Erikson, S., Alm, R., Kristenson, H. (1984): In Bile Acids in Hepatobiliary and Gastrointestinal Disease. IRL Press, Oxford, p. 127

4. Rickers, H., Christensen, M., Arnfeld, T., Dige, U., Hess Taysen., E. (1982): Scand.J.Gastroenterol. 17, 565

5. Tobiassen, P., Boeryd, B. (1980): Scand. J. Gastroenterol. 15, 657

6. Campbell, C.B., McGuffie, C., Powell, L.W., Roberts, R.K., Stewart, A.W. (1978): Digest. Diseases 23, 599

Reprints to:

Prof. Dr. Ellen Schmidt
Abt. Gastroenterologie u.Hepatologie
Zentrum Innere Medizin u.Dermatologie
Med. Hochschule Hannover
Konstanty-Gutschow-Str. 8

D - 3000 Hannover 61
FRG

4

On the Recognition of Hepatotoxic Side Effects of Cyclosporin A (CyA) After Liver Transplantation (LTX)

E. SCHMIDT[1], F.W. SCHMIDT[1], K. WONIGEIT[2], P. NEUHAUS[2],
R. PICHLMAYR[2], M. BURDELSKI[3], with technical assistance of:
J. LOBERS[1], P. MAHERSTEDT[1], S. OHLENDORF[1]
and R. RAUPACH[1]

*Abt. Gastroenterologie und Hepatologie, Zentrum Innere Medizin und Dermatologie
[1], Klinik für Abdominal- und Transplantations-Chirurgie, Sentrum Chirurgie
[2], Abt. für Nieren- und Stoffwechsel-Erkrankungen, Zentrum Kinderheilkunde
und Humangenetik
[3], Medizinische Hochschule Hannover, F.R.G.*

Zusammenfassung

1. Das Enzym-Muster im Serum bei Cyclosporin-A-Hepato-
   toxicität zeigt Zeichen von Leberzellschädigung und
   Cholestase. Keine der nur mäßig erhöhten Enzym-Aktivi-
   täten korreliert signifikant mit dem gleichzeitig ge-
   messenen Cyclosporin-A-Spiegel im Blut.

2. Mit Hilfe der Diskriminanz-Analyse kann die Cyclo-
   sporin-A-Hepatotoxicität durch die Bestimmung von
   ASAT, ALAT, GLDH, LDH und GGT im Serum erkannt und von
   anderen Komplikationen nach Leber-Transplantation mit
   einer 80 %igen Treffsicherheit unterschieden werden.

3. Das Enzym-Muster bei lebertoxischen Cyclosporin-A-
   Wirkungen kann am ehesten mit dem bei Sepsis und bei
   Störungen des Galle-Abflusses verwechselt werden,
   weniger mit dem Bild bei akuten Abstoßungs-Reaktionen
   und gar nicht mit dem Muster der akuten Durchblutungs-
   Störungen der Leber.

4. Die Zuverlässigkeit der enzymatischen Befunde für
   Diagnose und Differential-Diagnose ist bei allen
   komplexen pathologischen Zuständen eingeschränkt.
   Dennoch reicht sie in der Regel aus, um eine Ent-
   scheidungshilfe für die Therapie zu bieten.

The nephrotoxic side effects of CyA have not seriously
hindered its successful application as immunosuppressant
after renal transplantation. Neither will the hepatotoxic effects of high CyA levels offset the therapeutical
advantages of the drug after liver grafting (1,2,3,4,5).
The question is, how to detect CyA hepatotoxicity and to
discriminate it from other complications after LTX, which
may require a different, even opposite treatment, such as
e.g. septicemia or acute rejection of the graft or
biliary obstruction.
We tried to solve this problem by means of enzyme determinations in serum (6).

Material and Methods
86 patients, 1 - 58 years of age, 38 men, 32 women,
16 children, who have survived after LTX (1972-83) between one week and more than 8 years. Determination of 8
enzymes in serum, according to (7), daily, weekly or in
longer intervals, depending on the clinical requirements.

Results and discussion
251 episodic or more permanent alterations of the enzyme
pattern in serum were observed. On the basis of clinical
signs and symptoms, of macroscopic and microscopic
morphological and imaging findings, of biochemical and
microbiological, these altered patterns were assigned to
main causes. These are listed on Table 1.
Besides the first and largest group, which comprises 75
more or less pronounced and typical immediate postoperative enzyme peaks, due to the disturbed perfusion of
the transplanted liver, there were 61 episodes, which
remained either unspecified or too complex for simple
classification. Both groups are left out of consideration
here.
The remaining diagnoses are, however, also not always as
clear or typical, as one might assume; frequently the
picture has multiple causes or is shrouded by therapeutical interferences.

Table 1 :   Enzyme elevations in serum after liver
transplantation

Predominant cause	Number
Postoperative perfusion deficiency	75
Acute rejection	32
Postoperative bile drainage problems	15
Septicemia	12
Cyclosporin A hepatotoxicity	10
Acute vascular failure to the liver	9
Chronic rejection (typical)	17
Cytomegaly (CMV) hepatitis	7
Tumor recurrence	5
Vanishing bile duct syndrome	5
Acute viral hepatitis	3
Multiple or unspecified	61

The first 5 complications appear is a rule in the early
postoperative period, the second 5 belong rather to the
later course. CyA overtreatment occurs chiefly after the
replacement of the parenteral by the oral application of
the drug, despite serial determinations of CyA levels in
blood and individual dosage. Unknown factors, arising
from absorption, impaired liver function and constitu-
tional metabolic peculiarities seem to distort the relationship between dose and blood level of CyA and between
blood level and overt hepatotoxicity.
Above 800 µg/l CyA in blood, there is no correlation
between the CyA level and the activity of any individual
enzyme activity in serum ($r \blacktriangleleft 0.1$). Therefore the serial
determinations of CyA levels are indeed necessary for the
monitoring of the immunosuppressive effect but insuffi-
cient to predict hepatotoxicity.

Fig. 1 shows the enzyme patterns in serum in 4 complications of the early postoperative period, as compared
to that of CyA hepatotoxicity. In the upper part, it can

be seen that in acute rejections and in septicemia most
enzymes are higher elevated than in CyA toxicity. In
addition septicemia stands out for its high LDH and low
CHE activity.

In acute vascular disturbances of the liver, lower left,
the cell enzymes are higher by an order of magnitude than
in all other conditions, including the indicators of
cholestasis, which is peculiar for the transplanted
liver. The biliary occlusions, lower right, shows the
typical pattern.

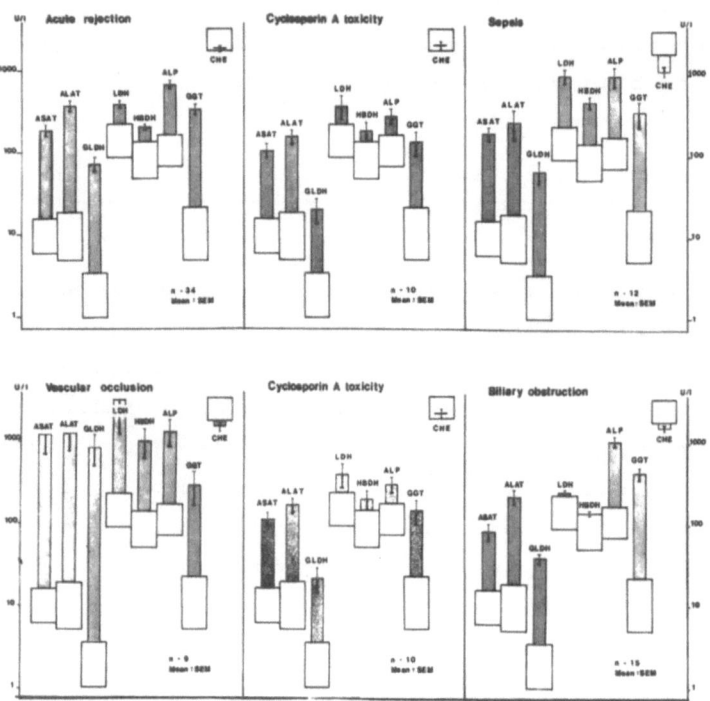

Fig. 1: Enzyme patterns in serum after liver transplantation. Early postoperative period: Differential
diagnosis of CyA hepatotoxicity.
ASAT = aspartate aminotransferase (E.C. 2.6.1.1);
ALAT = alanin aminotransferase (E.C. 2.6.1.2);
GLDH = glutamate dehydrogenase (E.C. 1.4.1.3);
LDH = lactate dehydrogenase (E.C. 1.1.1.27);
HBDH = alpha-hydroxybutyrate dehydrogenase (LDH
isoenzyme H_4); ALP = alkaline phosphatase (E.C.
3.1.3.1); GGT = gamma-glutamyl transferase (E.C.
2.3.2.2); CHE = cholinesterase (E.C. 3.1.1.8)

In Fig. 2 the enzyme pattern of CyA toxicity is confron-
ted to 4 patterns from the later course after liver
transplantation. The predominance of cholestasis is
conspicuous. It increases from CMV hepatitis via tumor
recurrence and typical chronic rejection to the syndrome
of vanishing bile ducts.

Although the differences of the patterns can be discerned,
it is conceivable that doubts arise, if by simple looking
at these pictures of enzymes patterns a significant
contribution to clinical differential diagnosis may be
achieved. In fact, even significant differences between
the mean values can be missing, e.g. between CyA toxicity
and CMV hepatitis. On the other hand there are as many as
6 significant differences of single enzymes and simple
enzyme ratios between CyA toxicity and vascular
occlusions or septicemia.

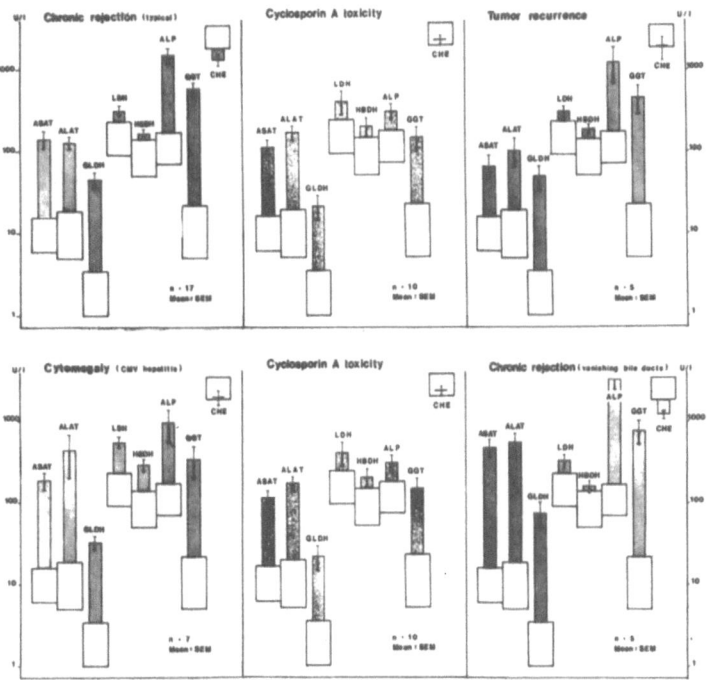

Fig. 2: Enzyme patterns in serum after liver transplanta-
        tion. Later course: Differential diagnosis of
        CyA hepatotoxicity. Abbreviations see Fig. 1.

Taking into account the variable severity of the respective complications and their sometimes rapid time course, which lead to a wide variation of the findings in individual cases, the value of significant differences of means must not be overestimated.

Rather, it would be preferable to try to substantiate mathematically the process which one attempts mentally every day, based on personal experience and memory, namely, to recognize and classify the patterns as wholes.

Table 2 shows the results of a multivariate discriminant analysis of the 5 diagnoses, which have the greatest significance in the early postoperative period. The logarithms of the enzyme activities have been used and redundant parameters have been identified and eliminated: these have been HBDH, ALP and CHE. With the remaining profile of 5 enzymes the overall reclassification amounted to 70 %. CyA toxicity is recognized best (80 %), in 10 % each it is misclassified as septic or biliary in origin. Vice versa, one case each of septicemia, biliary obstruction and acute rejection are erraneously classified as CyA toxicity.

With respect to the prevalence of CyA toxicity in the collective (o.16), the predictive value of the diagnosis "CyA toxicity" is o.73, the predictive value of the diagnosis "no CyA toxicity" is 0.96. The question if these predictive values are sufficient to provide, if need be, the basis for the possibly grave decision to reduce the dose of CyA or even change the immunosuppressant, cannot be answered in a positive way. At present, the numbers of patients investigated are to small, the CyA determination by RIA includes too many cross-reacting ill-defined metabolites, and the analysis of the enzymatic findings is frequently impeded by the superposition of multiple pathogenetic factors. Nevertheless, these preliminary results appear promising enough to proceed on this way.

Table 2 : Enzyme pattern in serum after liver transplantation (Discriminant analysis by log activities of the following enzymes: ASAT - ALAT - GLDH - LDH - GGT)

Classification:			(predicted group)			
Actual group	n	(1)	(2)	(3)	(4)	(5)
1 Cyclosporin A	10	8	0	1	0	1
toxicity		80	0	10	0	10 %
2 Acute vascular	9	0	7	1	1	0
failure		0	78	11	11	0 %
3 Septicemia	11	1	1	7	2	0
		9	9	64	18	0 %
4 Acute	18	1	0	3	11	3
rejection		6	0	17	61	17 %
5 Biliary	15	1	0	0	3	11
obstruction		7	0	0	20	73 %

Total	63	Correct classification	70 %

Summary and conclusions

1. The enzyme pattern in serum from CyA hepatotoxicity shows signs of cell damage as well as of cholestasis. None of the only moderately elevated enzyme activities correlates significantly with the concomitant CyA level in blood.

2. Cyclosporin A hepatotoxicity can be detected and dis-criminated from other early complications after liver transplantation by the determination of ASAT, ALAT, GLDH, LDH and GGT correct classification in 80 % by discrimi-nant analysis.

3. CyA hepatotoxicity may be confused mainly with septicemia and biliary obstruction, less likely with acute rejection and not with acute vascular failure.

4. The reliability of the enzymatic findings is impaired in all complex pathological conditions, but, as a rule, it is sufficient to be helpful in therapeutic decision making.

References

1. Hows, J.M. et al (1983). Brit.J.Haematol.54, 69-78

2. Powles, R.L.et al (1983). Lancet II, 1327-1331

3. Schade, R.R.et al (1983). Gastroenterology 84, 1298

4. Klintmalm,G.B.G.et al (1981). Transplantation 32,
   488 - 489

5. Wonigeit,K. et al (1983). Transplant.Proc. 15,
   Suppl. 1, 2586 - 2591

6. Schmidt, E. and F.W.: 11th Internat.Symp.Clin.
   Enzymol. 1984

7. Recommendations of GSCC: J.Clin.Chem.clin.Biochem.8,
   658, (1970)

Reprints to:

Prof.Dr. Ellen Schmidt

Abt.Gastroenterologie u. Hepatologie

Med.Hochschule Hannover

Konstanty-Gutschow-Str. 8

D - 3000 Hannover 61, FRG

5

Plasma Renin Activity and Renal Function in Liver Cirrhosis Before and After Liver Transplantation

A. ARMBRECHT, R. BRUNKHORST, Ch. BRÖLSCH, H. LIEBAU, K.M. KOCH, R. PICHLMAYR and K. KÜHN

Div. Nephrology, Dept. Internal Medicine and Dept. Abdominal and Transplantation Surgery, Hannover Medical School, Hannover, F.R.G.

Zusammenfassung

Bei 6 Patienten mit Leberzirrhose korrelierte eine hohe Plasma-Renin-Aktivität vor Lebertransplantation mit einem postoperativ ungünstigen Verlauf der glomerulären Filtrationsrate im Gegensatz zu 9 Patienten mit einer normalen Plasma-Renin-Aktivität. Von daher könnte eine hohe Plasma-Renin-Aktivität vor Lebertransplantation von prognostischer Bedeutung sein für den postoperativen Verlauf der Nierenfunktion.

Introduction

End stage liver cirrhosis is often associated with detoriation of renal function. IWATSUKI et al (1) reported that in patients with hepatorenal syndrome normalizing of glomerular filtration rate was observed after LTX. In one of the three described cases a high plasma renin activity was measured prior LTX. We investigated renal outcome after LTX in relation to the plasma renin activity prior to and after LTX in 15 patients with liver cirrhosis.

Methods

In 15 patients with liver cirrhosis the following parameters were determined prior to LTX and 1-2 days, 8-10 days and 28-30 days after LTX:

31

1. Plasma renin activity (PRA)
2. Creatinine clearance (C_{Cr})
3. Serum sodium concentration (S_{Na})
4. Urinary sodium concentration (U_{Na})

Prior LTX, in every patient diretic therapy was stopped
for at least 72 hrs before measurement of the parameters
was performed. Cyclosporin therapy with monitoring of
plasma levels was started 6 hrs prior to LTX and continued after LTX. In all patients mean arterial blood
pressure was above 90 mm Hg and central venous pressure
was above 5 cm H_2O prior to LTX.

Results

Regarding PRA prior to LTX two groups of patients could
be distinguished:
1. Normal renin group (NRG)   (table 1)
2. High renin group (HRG)

In the high renin group PRA was still elevated after LTX.
In the normal renin group PRA remained at a normal level
after LTX (table 1). Creatinine clearances showed no
significant differences prior to LTX in both groups.
8 - 10 days after LTX there was a significant decrease
of creatinine clearances in the high renin group in
contrast to the normal renin group (table 1). Serum
sodium concentration was lower in the high renin group
prior to LTX (table 1). Urinary sodium concentration
significantly decreased 8 - 10 days after LTX in the
high renin group.

The mean arterial blood pressure was comparable in both
groups prior to and after LTX. In the high renin group
all patients except one died within 30 days after LTX,
while eight patients from nine of the normal renin
group survived (table 1).

Table 1: NRG = normal renin group, HRG = high renin group. Plasma renin activity (PRA), creatinine clearance (C_{Cr}), serum sodium concentration (S_{Na}) and urinary sodium concentration (U_{Na}) in patients with liver cirrhosis before and after liver transplantation (LTX). In the HRG only one patient survived within 28-30 days after LTX, in the NRG eight patients survived.

		Before LTX	After LTX		
			1 - 2 days	8 - 10 days	28 - 30 days
P R A	NRG	2.7± 0.67 (n=8)	1.4± 0.43 (n=9)	1.6± 0.51 (n=9)	2.5± 1.06 (n=8)
ng/ml/h	HRG	13.2± 2.10 (n=5)	19.6± 5.23 (n=6)	16.0± 9.47 (n=6)	17.1 (n=1)
C c r	NRG	135.5±17.0 (n=8)	57.9±15.6 (n=9)	116.8+18.6 (n=9)	100.5±13.3 (n=8)
ml/min	HRG	94.2± 6.5 (n=5)	17.7+ 8.7 (n=6)	37.2+11.3 (n=6)	35 (n=1)
S N a	NRG	138.6± 1.07 (n=8)	142.2+ 1.53 (n=9)	136.4+ 1.70 (n=9)	137.1+ 1.57 (n=8)
mval/l	HRG	130.2+ 2.0 (n=5)	142.8+ 2.12 (n=6)	140.0+ 2.25 (n=6)	135 (n=1)
U N a	NRG	65.5+15.7 (n=8)	108.8+11.8 (n=9)	72.0+15.7 (n=9)	110.0+77.5 (n=8)
mval/l	HRG	62.6+14.4 (n=5)	100.3+19.4 (n=6)	16.8+ 4.0 (n=6)	19.0 (n=1)

Discussion

Since our results demonstrate, that there are significant
differences in renal function of patients with liver
cirrhosis after LTX, renal failure has to be considered
regarding prognosis of these patients : in the high
renin group renal failure was one of the major factors
contributing to the high mortality; liver failure was
seen in the minority (2/6) of these patients. The
reason for the elevated PRA prior to LTX in this group
of six patients is not clear. Diuretics were not given
in the period of PRA determination prior to LTX.
However, a prolonged effect of earlier intensive
diuretic treatment can not be excluded (2). In addition
diminished removal rate of renin by the cirrhotic
liver (3), a low effective blood volume (4) or a low
serum concentration as stimuli for renin secretion (5)
have to be considered. One can assume that persistent
high PRA followed by an intrarenal angiotension II
activation contributes to the developement of renal
failure after LTX in these patients.

References

1. Iwatsuki, S., Popovtzer, M.M., Cormann, J.L.,
   Ishikawa, M., Putman, C.W., Katz, F.H., Starzl, T.E.
   (1973): Recovery from "Hepatorenal Syndrome" after
   orthotopic liver transplantation. New Eng. J. Med.
   289, 1155 - 1159

2. Wernze, H., Spech, H.J., Müller, G. (1978):
   Studies on the activity of the renin-angiotension-
   aldosterone system (RAAS) in patients with cirrhosis
   of the liver. Klin. Wochenschr. 56, 389 - 397

3. Wernze, H., Seki, A., Schneider, K.W., Jesse, R.
   (1972): Extraktion und Clearance von Renin bei
   Leberzirrhose. Klin. Wochenschr. 50, 302 - 310

4. Epstein, M., Levinson, R., Sancho, J., Haber, E.,
   Re, R. (1972): Characterization of the renin-
   aldosterone system in decompensated cirrhosis.
   Circ. Res. 41, 818 - 829

5. Brown, J.J., Davies, D.L., Lever, A.F., Robertson,J.S.
   (1965): Plasma renin concentration in human
   hypertension. Relationship between renin, sodium
   and potassium.
   Br. Med. J. 2, 144 - 148

Reprints to:

Prof. Dr. K. Kühn
Div. Nephrology, Dept. Internal Medicine
Hannover Medical School
Konstanty-Gutschow-Str. 8

D - 3000 Hannover 61
FRG

6

The Role of TC-99m-IDA-Scintiscanning in Neonatal Jaundice and After Surgical Treatment of Biliary Atresia

K.F. GRATZ, H. CREUTZIG, M. BURDELSKI and H. HUNDESHAGEN

Zentrum Radiologie, Abtl. Nuklearmedizin und spezielle Physik und Zentrum Kinderheilkunde und Humangenetik, Abtl. Kinderheilkunde II, pädiatrische Nieren- und Stoffwechselkrankheiten, Medizinische Hochschule, Hannover, F.R.G.

Introduction

Cholescintigraphic agents are cleared by one of the separate carrier-mediated processes located at the sinosuidal site of the hepatocyte (CHERVU et al. 1982). This carrier mediated transport is impeded by the competitive binding of various inhibitors whose transport depends on the same carrier and storage sites. Ic-99m-IDA-derivates have been shown to be inhibited by increasing serum bilirubin concentration which limits the clinical usefulness in prolonged jaundice (GREEN 1982, WEISSMANN et al. 1981).

Biliary visualization with IDA-derivates is consistently obtained when the bilirubin level is normal or slightly elevated. About 85 to 90 % of the radiotracer is excreted via the hepatobiliary system and is availiable for detection. As hepatocellular function is compromised and the bilirubin level increases, a greater proportion of the applied Tc-99m-IDA-derivate is excreated via the kidneys and less via the hepatobiliary route. Lengthening the alkyl chain on the benzene ring of the IDA molecule results in enhanced hepatobiliary excretion. Thus newer cholescintigraphic agents as Tc-99m-diisopropyl iminodiacetic acid (DISIDA) expects much of detectability of the gallblader, the hepatobiliary tree or bile leakage even in cases of hyperbilirubinemia.

A pilot study was undertaken to develop a diagnostic scheme for differention of prolonged neonate jaundice with cholescintigraphy. A second study was done to evaluate the diagnostic value of moderne IDA-imaging after surgical interventions.

Technique

After an intravenous injection of 40 MBq Tc-99m-DISIDA, serial scintiphotos yield a dynamic representation of hepatobiliary function. The studies were performed in the supine position under a gamma camera equipped with a high sensitivity collimator and linked to a dedicated mini-computer. It is essential to obtain delayed views until fully hepatic excretion of the tracer in cases of possible biliary leakage or up to a maximum of 30 hr in the absence of gut visualization.

Patient selection

Diagnostic problems has been arised in 10 patients with neonatal jaundice. To confirm or to exclude the diagnosis of biliary leakage 66 patients were scintiscanned in the postoperative phase.

Results

Figure 1 demonstrats normal hepatobiliary DISIDA-kinetic in spite of hyperbilirubinemia due to a cephalhaematoma.

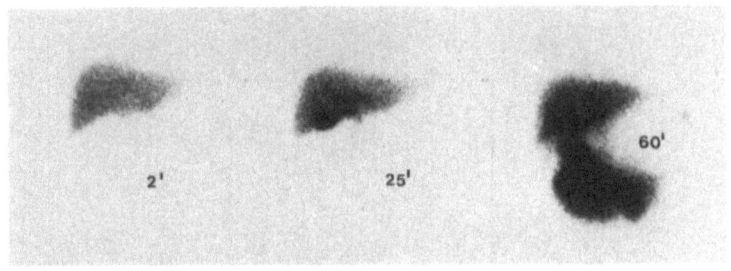

Fig. 1: Normal Tc-99m-DISIDA kinetic in a case of
        Cephalhaematoma

No or little renal excretion, gallbladder and biliary tree
visualization and early (up to 45 minutes p.i.) evidence
of intestinal activity are the conditions for normal bile
flow.

DISIDA-excretion is delayed in cases with hepatocellular
damage. In neonatal hepatitis gallbladder visualization
and intestinal activity is evident. Only in severe cases
it may be difficult to demonstrate bile flow into the
small bowel. Delayed views and computerizised image preparation are necessary (figure 2).

As long as some degree of bile flow into the intestine
is detectable, the presence of complete extrahepatic
biliary atresia is excluded (figure 2).

As figure 3 and 4 are demonstrating Tc-99m-DISIDA-imaging
is able to discriminate complete from partial atresia
and hypoplasia from atresia or hepatitis. Absence of left
or right biliary tree or gallbladder is typical for
partial atresia. In hypoplasia of the intrahepatic bile
ducts it is impossible to visualizise the biliary tree in
spite of timely evidence of intestinal activity.

After hepatic portoenterostomy, cholecystoenterostomy or
hepatic transplantation demonstrable bile flow via the
anastomosis excludes obstruction. In the early postoperative phase cholescintigraphy is employed for detec-

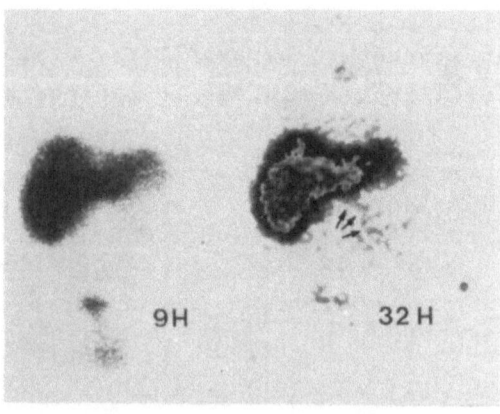

Fig. 2: Delayed visualization of intestinal activity in
        severe hepatocellular disease

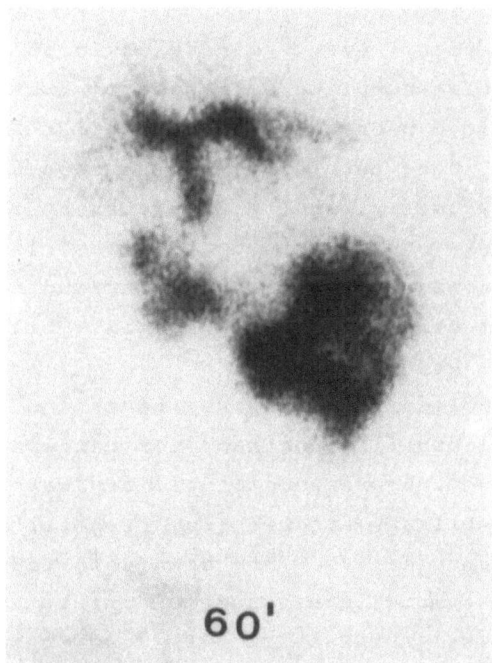

Fig. 3: Partial extrahepatic atresia: Incomplete
atresia of the pancreatic part of the bile
duct, atresia of the gallbladder and cystic
duct.

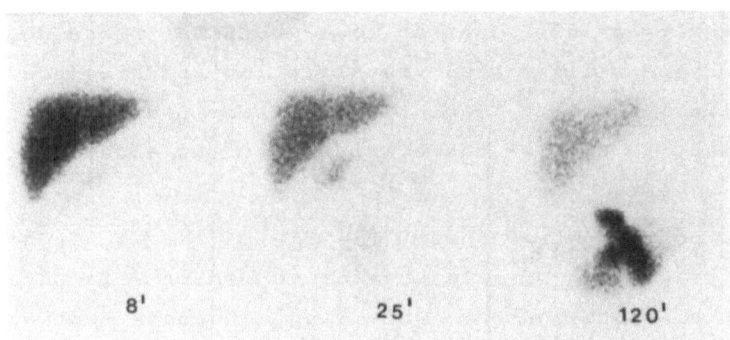

Fig. 4: Intrahepatic biliary hypoplasia: No visualization
of the biliary tree and gallbladder but early
presence of intestinal activity.

tion of bile leakage. 19 of 66 patients have had bile
leakage demonstrated by cholescintigraphy and confirmed
by relaparatomy. Only in 2 cases bile leakage was over-
looked.

Discussion

In Western Germany, every year 40 children were born with
biliary atresia. Complete extrahepatic ductal obstruction
in the jaundiced neonate is an indication for surgical
intervention. Long-term follow-up studies have indicated
significantly better results when surgery is performed
before 10 weeks of age. Frequently, the clinical course,
closed needle biopsy, ultrasonography and in vitro
laboratory studies cannot differentiate biliary atresia
from neonatal hepatitis.

Therefore, cholescintigraphy may be the only procedure
capable of eliminating the need for unnecessary surgery
by documenting the presence of biliary patency. For
differention biliary atresia from neonatal hepatitis, an
overall accuracy of 100 % has been reported (DAUMERIE
et al. 1983) even without duodenal intubation and juice
collection (TWEI-SHIUN et al. 1984) or phenobarbital
premedication (MAJD et al. 1981).

The aim of the present study was to assess the ability
of the Tc-99m-IDA-scan for the differential diagnosis of
neonatal cholestasis. It seems possible to differentiate
five entities in respect to Tc-99m-DISIDA-uptake, gallbladder and biliary tree visualization and presence of
intestinal activity (Table 1). Further investigations are
necessary to confirm the clinical use and accuracy of the
given scheme.

In the postoperative phase, Tc-99m-IDA-imaging is done in
order to exclude bile leakage or to demonstrate patency
of the portoenterostomy. This study suggests that non-
invasive cholescintigraphy can detect bile leakage
accuratly (90 % sensitivity, 100 % specifity). Further
differentiation of the leakage side is possible
(GRATZ et al. 1982).

Table 1: Differential diagnose of neonatal cholestasis
         with Tc-99m-DISIDA

Tc-99m-DISIDA-imaging :	uptake	gallbladder biliary tree	gut activity
Prehepatic disease	normal	demonstrable	timely
Hepatocellular disease	decreased	demonstrable	delayed
Biliary hypoplasia	normal	failure	timely
Partial biliary atresia	normal	partial failure	timely
Complete biliary atresia	normal/ decreased	failure	absent

References

1. Chervu, L.R., Nunn, A.D., and Loberg, M.D. (1982).
   Radiopharmaceuticals for hepatobiliary imaging.
   Sem.Nucl.Med. 12, 5-17

2. Daumerie,C., Pauwels, S., Otte,J.B., Buts,J.P. and
   Piret, L. (1983). Tc-99m-Diethyl-IDA-imaging in
   neonatal jaundice. Annual Meeting of the Societe Belge
   de Medicine Nucleaire, 26.11.1983 in Brussels

3. Gratz,K.F., Creutzig, H., Brölsch, C. et al. (1982).
   Choleszintigraphie bei Verdacht auf Galleleck ; In:
   R.Höfer, H.Bergmann (ed.): Radioaktive Isotope in
   Klinik und Forschung, Egermann, Wien, 189-194

4. Green,M. (1982). Developing a new hepatobiliary
   imaging agent. Diagnostic Imaging 6, 34-38

5. Majd,M., Reba, R.C., and Altman, R.P. (1981). Effect
   of Phenobarbital on Tc-99m-IDA scintigraphy in the
   evaluation of neonatal jaundice. Sem.Nucl.Med. 11,
   194-204

6. Twei-Shiun,J., Wu,C., Ho,Y., Huang,B., and Lu,C.
   (1984).Diagnosis of obstructive jaundice in infants:
   Tc-99m DISIDA in duodenal juice. J.Nucj.Med.25,360-363

7. Weissmann,H.S., Sugarman,L.A., and Freeman, L.M.
   (1981). The clinical role of Tc-99m iminodiacetic
   acid cholescintigraphy. In: L.M. Freeman, H.S. Weissmann (ed.): Nuclear Medicine Annual 1981, Raven Press,
   New York, 35-89

Reprints to:

K.F. Gratz, MD
Dept. Nuclear Medicine
Medical High School of Hannover
Konstanty-Gutschow-Str. 8

D - 3000 Hannover 61
FRG

Chronic Active Hepatitis

7

Hepatitis B versus Dioxin (TCDD) in the Pathogenesis of Excess Primary Liver Cell Carcinoma in Viet Nam[1],[2]

C. JERUSALEM[3], K. KUBAT[4] and W. ELING[3]

[1]*In commemoration of Professor Ton That Tung, famous surgeon and scientist, previous chief of the Viet Duc Hospital, Hanoi (S.R. of Viet Nam) who raised and maintained the discussion on the long-term effects of 2,3,7,8-tetrachlorodibenzo-p-dioxin (TCDD)*
[2]*Party supported by Grant TSD-M-044-NL of the Commission of the European Communities*
[3]*Department of Cytology & Histology,* [4]*Department of Pathology of the Catholic University of Nijmegen, The Netherlands*

Zusammenfassung

In Viet Nam stieg in den letzten Jahren die Häufigkeit des primären Leberzellkarzinoms (HCC) sprunghaft an, besonders in den Gebieten, die während den II.Indochina- krieges intensiv mit dem mit Dioxin (TCDD) verunreinigten Herbizid "Agent Orange" besprüht worden waren. Da nur bei älteren Karzinomträgern eine Korrelation mit persistieren- der viraler Hepatitis B nachzuweisen war und da in Viet Nam die sonst in tropischen Ländern als weitere Hauptverursacher des HCC angesehenen Faktoren wie Myko- toxine oder Schistosomiasis und Opisthorchosis fehlen, wird die Rolle des TCDD in der Genese des HCC vor allem bei jüngeren Patienten diskutiert. TCDD könnte entweder direkt auf Grund seiner Hepatotoxizität oder indirekt als "promoting Agent" wirken, das im Rahmen der Zweiphasen- theorie nur die morphologische Manifestation einer voran- gehenden malignen Transformation induziert.

During the second Indochina war, mainly between 1961 and 1970, U.S.A. military aircrafts sprayed 59 million kilo- grams of the anti-plant ingredient "Agent Orange" (respectively ((-2,4-D; 2,4,5-T)) N-butylic- 2,4-di

---

Key words: Hepatocellular carcinoma; Viet Nam; Agent Orange, Dioxin

((and 2,4,5-tri-)) chlorophenoxy acetic acid), 26 million
kilograms of "Agent White" (2,4-D and picloram) and 11
million kilograms of "Agent Blue" (dimethyl-arsenic
((-cacodylic)) over selected areas of the central and
southern regions of Viet Nam (WESTING 1984). About 10 per
cent of the dense inland forests and 40 per cent of the
mangrove habitat was destroyed. In relation to the population in some areas up to 9.73 kilograms per capita
were dispensed.
The phenoxy herbicides (2,4-D, 2,4,5-T) also contained
at least a total amount of 172 kilograms of 2,3,7,8-
tetrachlorodibenzo-p-dioxin (TCDD) as an impurity.
"Dioxin" (TCDD) is probably the most toxic man-made substance known, producing changes in various organs, metabolic alterations and is suggested to initiate hepatocellular carcinoma (KOCIBA et al. 1979, SUGAR et al.
1979).

Studies of TON THAT TUNG (1975) on Vietnamese populations
have produced suggestive evidence of an increasing excess
of hepatocellular carcinoma (HCC), particularly among
those populations who had been exposed to military
herbicides for several years. In view of the general
importance of the long-term effects on man of TCDD
contaminated herbicides the present study compares the
morphology of HCC of Viet Namese populations who had
been exposed, with those not exposed to military phenoxy
herbicides.

Material and methods
Two groups of intraoperative wedge biopsies and post
mortem specimens of HCC were compared (see Table 1):
1) 33 cases of HCC in patients, who had been exposed to
   fall outs of Agent Orange and/or stood in TCDD
   contaminated areas (respectively the war zones I and
   III+IV, subgroups 1a and 1b) for several years during
   the 1960's and 1970's.

Table 1: Hepatitis B in Viet Namese patients with
         hepatocellular carcinoma

		HCC	patients	from
Region (Viet Nam)	South		North	South
Group	1a	1b	2	controls[1]
War zone	I	III+IV	-	-
Number of patients	16	17	28	28
TCDD contact	yes	yes	no	no
Age (years)	32-59	27-53	35-56	16-58
Collected between	1975-79	1977-82	1975-78	1976-78
HBs positive by Shikata (%)	75.0	35.3	57.1	60.7
immune assay (%)	not done	1981:29.4%	not done	not done
History of malaria (P. falciparum (%))	16.5	23.5	7.1	100

[1] Deaths of P. falciparum malaria

2) 28 cases of HCC of patients from the northern regions
   of Viet Nam and thus not subjected to military
   herbicides.

Non-tumorous livers of 18 patients who died of P. falciparum malaria served as control. (For age of patients
and period of collection of specimens see Table 1).

Histological sections of paraffin-embedded material were
stained with haematoxylin and eosin, Goldner's trichrome,
PAS and for demonstration of hepatitis B surface antigen
(HBsAg) according to SHIKATA et al.(1974). Since 1981
hepatitis B was also determined by an immune assay. These
figures largely correlate with histological findings
(Table 1).

Results

The microscopic appearance of hepatic neoplasma did not
differ among group 1 and 2. Most tumors were of the
trabecular, pseudoglandular and occasionally of the clear
cell type. The pleomorphic cytological variant was
infrequent.
Macronodular liver cirrhosis was the usual finding in

association with HCC. In the liver of patients who had been exposed to military phenoxy herbicides (group 1), however, there was an obvious coincidence of the neoplastic change with a macronodular lesion which resembled respectively the focal nodular hyperplasia, or "enzyme altered" foci, and of changes suggestive of a preneoplastic lesion. Presumable preneoplastic cells were those large dysplastic hepatocytes with either bizarre hyperchromatic nuclei, or with more than 2 nuclei, with occasionally large nucleoli, and either a basophilic cytoplasm or a rough endoplasmic reticulum condensed around the nucleus. Occasionally, in the same liver the presumptive preneoplastic change resembled the type of the carcinoma.

In cells of the hyperplastic nodules HBs antigen could never be demonstrated. Shikata-positive cells were restricted to the original liver tissue which had frequently been displaced to the nodular periphery. Occasionally Kupffer cells had phagocytozed a Shikata-positive substance.

The coincidence of HCC with HBs antigen was rather high in group 1a and 2 (respectively 75 % and 57 %; Table 1), while it was low in group 1b (35 %). However, the association of HCC with HBsAg was largely age-dependent, except of group 1b. Of the 10 patients younger than 39 years, 8 were negative for HBsAg and only 2 positive. Among the 39 patients aged between 40 and 49 years 18 were negative and 21 positive, while only one negative case was found among the 12 patients who were older than 50 years. In patients younger than 39 years a striking difference had been noticed between those who had been exposed (6 negative, 1 positive for HBsAg) or not (2 positive, 1 negative) to phenoxy herbicides.

Discussion

A variety of factors has been suggested to be involved in hepatocellular carcinogenesis (HCCis). In temperate

zones, in approximately 65 % to 70 % postnecrotic cirrhosis, mainly due to persistant viral hepatitis (PVHB),
appears to precede HCC. The excess of HCC in various
tropical countries is suggested, too, to be related to
PVHB, although HCC and liver cirrhosis arise almost
simultaneously and these patients die with their tumor
without having had any history of liver cirrhosis
(ALPERT et al. 1969).

Other etiological factors that are recognized are the
parasites Opisthorchis viverrini and Schistosoma
japonicum, as well as dietary toxins, such as aflatoxin,
sterigmatoxin and cycasin. In Viet Nam, however, opisthorchosis and schistosomiasis are unknown and dietary myco-
toxins appear to play a minor role because the main
source of aflatoxin, the ground nut, is a quite uncommon
food product. HCC was also not correlated to previous
attacks of P. falciparum malaria (Table 1).

A rather puzzling observation is the difference in tumor-
associated HBsAg particularly between group 1a and 1b.
The propagation of hepatitis B is a common result of
disasterous hygienic conditions during war times. Since
HBsAg positivity was most frequently correlated with HCC
in older patients, the excess of liver tumors could be
explained with an increase in frequency of PVHB, whether
these patients had been exposed or not to phenoxy herbicides. In contrast, the majority of the younger patients
did not suffer from PVHB, suggesting other etiological
factors to be involved in HCCis.

It is well recognized that secondary to liver injury the
hepatic parenchymal cells undergo compensatory hyperplasia. Following continuous injury secondary to specific
infections, inborn metabolic disorders, dietary myco-
toxins, alcohol and industrial chemicals, this hyperplastic response is mainly focal, and subsequent development of hepatocellular carcinoma is not necessarily
associated with a recognized carcinogen.

Recently as an alternative concept the two-stage process
of tumorigenesis has been proposed that distinguishes
between initiation and promotion (PITOT and SIRICA 1980).
The initiating factor is defined as an agent capable of
directly altering the genetic component of the cell. However, mere initiation by "incomplete" carcinogens,
causes only irreversible change but no neoplasm, unless
a promoting agent is applied. The promoting agent does
not directly interact with the genetic material but
effects its expression mainly by binding to cell surface
receptors. Recently, dioxin (TCDD) has been suggested to
be implicated in HCCis (JERUSALEM and KUBAT 1983). In
mice and rats the development of hyperplastic nodules
and HCC appeared to be TCDD dose dependent (KOCIBA et al.
1979) while in other experiments TCDD showed no initiating effect on carcinogenesis (SUGAR et al.1979), but
could act as a powerful promoting agent in HCCis
secondary to diethylnitrosamin combined with partial
hepatectomy (PITOT et al. 1980).
The majority of authors agree on a species-dependent
hepatoxicity of TCDD, that causes an unusual form of
injury particularly in rodents (GREIG et al. 1973,
MCCONNEL and MOORE 1979). Toxic metabolic disorders of
the liver have been registered, too, in industrial
workers who had been exposed to TCDD for several years
because of failures in chemical factories (MAY 1980,
PAZDEROVA-VEJLUPKOVA 1981).

In Viet Namese populations that had been exposed to
military phenoxy herbicides for long periods TCDD could
be implicated in HCCis in an indirect and direct manner:
in the case of an existing chronic liver injury (PVHB,
unspecific hepatitis) TCDD could act as an promoting
agent and/or due to its inherent hepatotoxicity,
aggravate and accelerate liver cell damage with the risk
of malignant mutation because of unphysiological
increased mitotic turn-over rates, and thus shortening

the latency period of HCCis. Since in addition signs of
exposure to TCDD include lassitude, impotence, nerve
disorders, abortation and teratogenetic disorders in
offsprings (SUN 1983) critical clinical studies of the
long-term effects of chlorinated dioxins are urgently
required, not only with respect of the victims of a
chemical warfare but also to populations who were the
dupe of accidents during production or application of
herbicides.

References

Alpert, H.E., Hutt, M.S.R. and Davidson, C.S. (1968).
    Hepatoma in Uganda: A study in geographis pathology.
    Lancet i, 1265-1267
Greig, J.B., Jones,G., Butler,W.H. and Barnes,J.M. (1973).
    Toxic effects of 2,3,7,8-tetrachlorodibenzo-p-dioxin.
    Food and Cosmetic Toxicology 11, 585-595
Hay, A. (1980). Chemical company suppresses dioxin
    report. Nature 284, 2
Jerusalem, C. and Kubat, K.(1983). Considerations ana-
    tomo-pathologiques du carcinome hépato-cellulaire chez
    les vietnamiens exposés aux phénoxy-herbicides mili-
    taires contaminés par la TCDD. In: Symposium Inter-
    national sur les herbicides et defoliants employes
    dans la guerre. Comité National d'Investigation,
    pp. 53-62, Hanoi
Kociba, R.J., Keyes,D.G., Beyer, J.E., Carreon, R.M.and
    Gehring, P.J. (1979). Long-term toxicologic studies
    of 2,3,7,8-tetrachlorodibenzo-p-dioxin (TCDD) in
    laboratory animals. Ann.N.Y.Acad. Sci.320, 397-404
McConnel,E.E. and Moore, J.A. (1979). Toxicopathology
    characteristics of the halogenated aromatic's.
    Ann. N.Y. Acad.Sci. 320, 138-150
Pazderova-Vejlupkova,A.J., Lukas,E., Nemcova, M.,
    Pickova, J. and Jirasek, L. (1981). The development
    and prognosis of chronic intoxication by tetra-chloro-
    dibenzo-p-dioxin in men.Arch.Environ.Health 36, 5-´ ˜

Pitot, H.C. and Sirica, A.E. (1980). The stages of
    initiation and promotion in hepatocarcinogenesis.
    Biochim.Biophys. Acta 605, 191-215

Pitot, H.C., Goldsworthy, T., Campbell, H.A. and
    Poland, A. (1980). Quantitative evaluation of the pro-
    motion by 2,3,7,8-tetrachlrodibenzo-p-dioxin of
    hepatocarcinogenesis from diethylnitrosamin. Cancer
    Res. 40, 3616-3620

Shikata, L., Uzawa, T., Joshiwara, N., Akatsuka, T. and
    Yamazaki, S. (1974). Staining methods of Australia
    antigen in paraffin sections. Detection of cytoplasmic
    inclusion bodies. Japan.J.Exp.Med. 44, 25-36

Sugar, J., Toth, K., Csuka, O., Gati, E. and Somfai-
    Relle, S. (1979). Role of pesticides in hepato-
    carcinogenesis. J.Toxicol.Environ.Health. 5, 183-191

Sun, M. (1983). Dioxins uncertain legacy. Science 219,
    468-469

Westing, A.H. (1984). Herbicides in war. The long-term
    ecological and human consequences. Taylor and Francis,
    London and Philadelphia.

Reprints to:

Prof.Dr.med. C.Jerusalem
Institut Zytologie und Histologie
Geert Groteplein N 21

6500 HB Nimegen
Netherlands

8

Assessment of Infectivity in Hepatitis B Virus Infected Individuals by Detection of HBV and Core Antigen in Serum

H. von WULFFEN, R. BREDEHORST, E. ZYZIK*
and W.H. GERLICH

Institut für Medizinische Mikrobiologie, Universität Hamburg, *Hygiene-Institut, Universität Göttingen

Zusammenfassung

Die vorliegende Studie befaßt sich mit dem Nachweis von HBV-DNA und Core-Antigen im Serum zur Beurteilung der Infektiosität bei Hepatitis-B-Virusinfektionen. Der HBV-DNA-Hybridisierungstest und der hier angewandte HBcAg-Test, der die Bestimmung von Core-Antigen im Serum in Gegenwart des homologen Antikörpers, des anti-HBc, ermöglicht, zeigten dabei ein hohes Maß an Übereinstimmung: Bei insgesamt 610 untersuchten HBsAg positiven Seren kam es nur in 2,6 % zu abweichenden Ergebnissen. Im einzelnen ergaben sich dabei folgende Befunde: In 228 HBeAg-positiven Seren ließ sich in 77 % der Fälle HBV-DNA nachweisen und in 72 % das Core-Antigen. In 213 anti-HBe-positiven Seren fand sich HBV-DNA in 9 und HBcAg in 10 Fällen. Von 169 HBsAg-positiven Seren, die weder HBeAg noch anti-HBe enthielten, zeigten 5 ein positives Ergebnis im HBV-DNA-Hybridisierungstest und 4 im HBcAg-Test.

Der Core-Ag-Test stellt somit eine wertvolle Ergänzung bzw. Alternative zum HBV-DNA-Hybridisierungstest bei der Beurteilung der Infektiosität dar. Weiterhin lassen beide Tests diesbezüglich deutliche Vorteile erkennen gegenüber dem HBeAg/anti-HBe-Testsystem. Außerdem scheint es so zu sein, daß der Nachweis von HBV-DNA bzw. Core-Ag in

HBeAg-negativen Seren mit oder ohne anti-HBe häufig mit
einer chronischen Hepatitis verknüpft ist.

The level of infectivity of HBsAg positive blood varies
widely. Many chronic carriers of the viral surface antigen do not have detectable HBV particles in their blood.
When HBV particles are present at high levels, a soluble
low molecular weight polypeptide, HBeAg, is usually
found in the serum of these patients. This HBeAg is a
part of the viral nucleoprotein and, like the HBsAg
20 nm particles, it is also a by-product of the viral
genome produced in excess of requirements for the formation of HBV particles. Currently, HBeAg in serum is considered to be an indirect marker of high infectivity.

Direct markers for complete infectious Dane particles are
the HBV associated endogenous DNA polymerase and,
recently, the HBV DNA itself. The latter can be detected
in serum specifically and sensitively by hybridization
with cloned and ^{32}P labelled HBV DNA (1). The detection
limit of the method which was used for this report is
10^6 genomes/ml. The method employed digestion of the sera
with proteinase, extraction of the DNA with phenol and
adsorption of the DNA to membrane filters.

Another way of detecting HBV particles in serum may be
an assay of the core antigen. HBcAg is, in contrast to
the afore mentioned HBsAg and HBeAg, usually not present
in serum as a soluble protein, but exclusively in the
core particle of the HBV. The difficulty of detecting
this antigen in the presence of its homologous antibody,
anti-HBc, has been overcome by a new technique that
allows detection of immune complexed antigens (2).
Briefly (figure 1), core particles are released from
Dane particles in serum by detergents and allowed to
form immune complexes with anti-HBc present in the serum
of HBV infected individuals. These immune complexes are
then precipitated by polyethylene glycol (PEG). The precipitated immune complexes are then dissociated by

thiocyanate (SCN$^-$), and subsequently adsorbed to polystyrene balls without prior removal of the chaotropic
ions. Thereby, HBcAg and anti-HBc are bound to the solid
phase independently of each other allowing subsequent
detection of HBcAg by ^{125}I marked anti-Hbc (3).

It was an open question whether the detection of core
antigen would correlate well with the presence of viral
DNA, for it is well known that HBV particles may be
devoid of DNA and a large excess of empty core particles
has been found in certain sera (4).

To study that correlation, different groups of HBsAg
positive sera were tested for the presence of HBcAg and
the results compared to those obtained in the HBV DNA
hybridization assay.

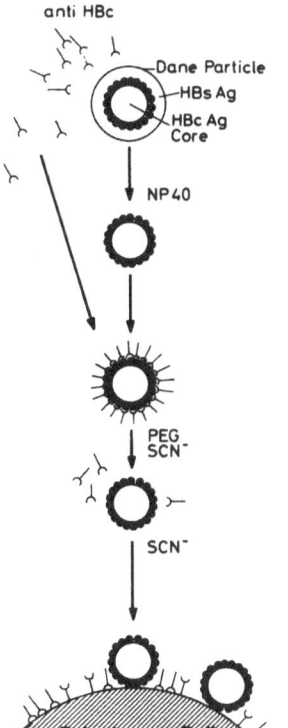

anti HBc

Dane Particle
HBs Ag
HBc Ag
Core

NP40

1. Release of core particles by
   NP40 treatment

2. Formation of immune complexes
   (ICs)

PEG
SCN$^-$

3. PEG-precipitation
4. Dissociation of ICs by
   3M thiocyanate

SCN$^-$

5. Adsorption under dissociating
   conditions

6. Determination of HBc Ag with
   ^{125}J - anti HBc

Polystyrene Ball

Figure 1: Detection of HBcAg from HBV particles in the
presence of anti-HBc

As seen in table 1, the qualitative results of the two
assays correlated very well: both tests were positive in
177 and negative in 417 cases out of a total of 610
tested sera. Deviating results were obtained in only 16
cases, i.e. in 2.6 % of the tested sera. A close quantitative correlation, however, between the concentration
of HBcAg and the amount of detected HBV DNA was not
observed. This suggests that the ratio of complete to
incomplete Dane particles is not constant in different
sera.

Table 1: Correlation of HBcAg and HBV DNA in 610 HBsAg
         positive sera.

		HBcAg	
		+	−
HBV DNA	+	177	12
	−	4	417

Of special interest was the correlation between the
e-antigen-antibody system and the more direct viral
markers: HBV DNA was found in 77 % and HBcAg in 72 % of
228 HBeAg positive sera, i.e. the HBcAg assay showed in
general a somewhat lower sensitivity than the HBV DNA
hybridization assay. For this reason, it was surprising
that three sera showed a positive result in the HBcAg
assay but no detectable HBV DNA. All three sera showed
positive DNA polymerase activity, two had high titres of
HBeAg, and two to the patients were known to have chronic
active hepatitis histologically. Whether the amount of
HBV was actually below the detection limit in these
cases or whether other reasons brought about the negative
results in the hybridization study remains open.

High HBeAg titres above 1: 128 in radioimmunoassay were
found in sera which contained HBV DNA and HBcAg. However,
lower HBeAg titres were not indicative of the presence or
absence of HBV DNA or HBcAg.

This is further underlined by the results obtained
from anti-HBe positive persons, i.e. a group that is
generally considered to be at low risk of transmitting
infection (5). In agreement with that expectation,
HBV DNA and HBcAg could not be detected in 105 anti-
HBe positive sera obtained from individuals at blood
donation. However, from 108 anti-HBe positive sera
selected from diagnostic samples on the basis of a
relatively high HBsAg content (➤ 5 µg/ml), 10 sera
were found to contain core antigen, 9 of them were
also positive for HBV DNA. Table 2 presents these cases
in more detail :   again the majority of these patients
suffered from chronic hepatitis. This finding confirmed previous observations that anti-HBe positive
sera may be infectious (6).

Finally, HBsAg positive sera were studied that were
negative both for HBeAg and anti-HBe. In 169 such sera
we found HBV DNA in 5 cases, 4 of which also had
detectable HBcAg. Again, four of these patients had
chronic hepatitis.

In conclusion, the HBcAg assay described above, allowing the detection of core antigen in serum in the
presence of its homologous antibody, shows a high
level of correlation with the HBV DNA hybridization
assay. It may thus serve as a valuable supplement to
this assay or as an alternative method were the HBV DNA
hybridization assay is not available. Both tests offer
more specific information than the HBeAg/anti-HBe system.
The detection of core antigen and/or HBV DNA in HBeAg
negative sera with or without anti-HBe seems to
correlate frequently with chronic liver disease.

Table 2: Diagnosis and markers of HBV particles in 10 HBsAg positive patients with <u>anti-HBe</u> Hepatitis B Virus (HBV) markers in serum

Case no.	Diagnosis	Anti-HBe (1/titer)	HBcAg (S:N ratio)	HBV DNA polymerase (pmol/ml x 10^2)	HBV DNA (genomes/ml)	HBsAg (µg/ml)
1	CAH	10^2	2.3	20.8	3×10^8	20
2	CAH	10^1	4.3	0.9	8×10^6	19
3	CAH	10^3	6.0	5.3	4×10^6	20
4	CAH	10^2	2.7	3.3	3×10^7	19
5	CAH	10^2	5.1	not tested	8×10^6	42
6	CPH	10^1	2.2	17.7	5×10^8	31
7	persistently elevated ALT	10^2	11.0	1.6	8×10^6	16
8	persistently elevated ALT	10^4	2.3	1.8	8×10^6	26
9	healthy HBsAg carrier	10^1	2.3	negative	negative	10
10	convalescent phase of acute HBV infection	10^0	2.1	negative	3×10^6	78

CAH = chronic active hepatitis, CPH = chronic persistent hepatitis, ALT = alanine amino-transferase, S : N ratio = ratio of cpm (counts per minute) of sample to cpm of negative control. Samples with S : N ratios 2.1 were considered to be positive in the HBcAg assay.

References

1. Berninger, M., Hammer, M., Hoyer, B., Gerin, J.L.
   (1982): An assay for the detection of the DNA genome
   of hepatitis B virus in serum. J. Med. Virol 9,
   57 - 68

2. Neurath, A. R., Strick, N., Baker, L., Krugman, S.
   (1982). Proc. Natl. Acad. Sci. USA 79, 4415 - 19

3. Bredehorst, R., von Wulffen, H., Granato, C.
   (1984). Quantitation of hepatitis B core antigen
   in serum in the presence of anti-HBc antibodies.
   Submitted for publication.

4. Alberti, A., Diana, S., Scullard, G.H.,
   Eddleston, A.L.W.F., Williams, R. (1978). Full
   and empty Dane particles in chronic hepatitis B
   virus infection: relation to hepatitis B e antigen
   and presence of liver damage. Gastroenterology 75,
   869 - 74

5. Eleftherio, U., Thomas, M.C., Heathcote, J.,
   Sherlock, S. (1975). Incidence and clinical
   significance of e antigen and antibody in acute
   and chronic clinical liver disease. Lancet 2,
   1171 - 1173

6. Berquist, K.R., Maynard, J.F., Murphy, B.L. (1976).
   Infectivity of serum containing HBsAg and antibody
   to e antigen.
   Lancet 1, 1026 - 1027

Reprints to:

Dr.med. H. von Wulffen
Institut für Mikrobiologie
Universität Hamburg
Martinistr. 52

D - 2000 Hamburg 20

9

Decreased Detoxification Capacity of the Liver in Chronic Active Hepatitis (Observations in 224 patients)

D. MÜTING[1], G. WINTER[2], J.F. KALK[1] and R. FISCHER[1]

[1]*Heinz Kalk-Klinik, Bad Kissingen, F.R.G.*
[2]*Leopoldina Hospital, Schweinfurt, F.R.G.*

Zusammenfassung

Bei 224 Patienten mit laparoskopisch und leberbioptisch gesicherter chronisch-aktiver Hepatitis (CAH) verschiedener Schweregrade wurden im Blut bzw. Plasma Ammoniak, freie Phenole und Indikan und im Harn die Ausscheidung an Harnstoff-N unter Standard-Diät meist im Rahmen von längeren Verlaufsuntersuchungen bestimmt.
Dabei zeigte sich eine signifikante Zunahme aller drei toxischer Eiweißmetaboliten parallel zur Zunahme der entzündlichen Aktivität und der portalen Hypertension.
Bei klinischer und morphologischer Besserung der CAH kam es auch zu einer signifikanten Abnahme von Ammoniak, Phenolen und Indikan im Blut, während sie bei Übergang in eine portale Hypertension deutlich zunahmen. Durch Lactulose, Bifidum-Milch und ammoniaksenkende Aminosäuren ließen sich sowohl psychische Veränderungen wie Depressionen und Aggressionen als auch toxische Eiweißmetaboliten im Blut günstig beeinflussen.

In follow-up controls of 650 patients with chronic active hepatitis (CAH) we noticed as well as WILDHIRT (1) considerable psychical disorders, mainly a tendency to depressions and aggressions which parallel more or less to the inflammatory activity of the liver.

The question came up whether decreased detoxification capacity of the liver may possibly appear in CAH. Already in 1969 we found a significant increase of plasma ammonia and free serum phenols in 60 patients with chronic hepatitis (2) . Meanwhile these analyses were performed in follow-up studies for years in chronic persistent hepatitis (CPH) and the different stages of CAH, in order to search for the relations between the morphological changes and disorders of the detoxification capacity in the liver. Furthermore, it is of interest, in how far those changes are influential by treatment and if they have a prognostic importance.

For this reason determinations of plasma ammonia were performed in 224 patients with laparoscopically and histologically proven CAH of different stages. The most important clinical, biochemical and morphological values are settled in our first communication (3) . Because of the shortness of time only the most important results should be mentiond.

First we touch the question of the behaviour of plasma ammonia, indican and free serum phenols of the different stages of chronic hepatitis on admission to hospital (fig. 1). In comparison with healthy adults, the plasma ammonia increases in form of a gauging graph from CPH up to CAH with cirrhotic transformation. The investigated values correspond to those in completely active liver cirrhosis without portal hypertension. In comparison with healthy adults the hyperammonemia is significant in CAH IIa, CAH IIb and CAH with transformation into cirrhosis.

Little steeper is the increase of free serum phenols. In part, phenols are bound in the liver on glucuronic acid or sulphuric acid and are excreted detoxified by the urine. Only free, thus non-bound serum phenols, are toxic. Their increase is as well significant in CAH IIa, CAH IIb and CAH with beginning cirrhosis. The cured, defectively cured, and improved patients show a significant decrease of plasma ammonia during the time of obser-

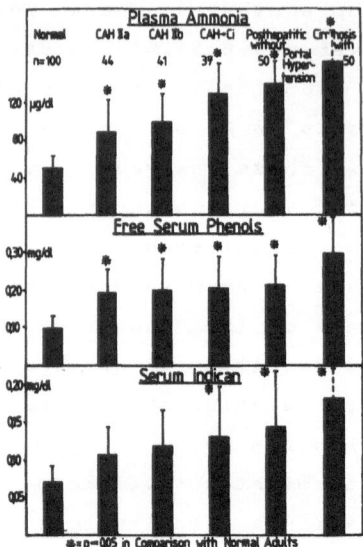

Fig. 1: Toxic protein metabolites (ammonia, free phenols
         and indican)in the blood of 224 patients with
         chronic active hepatitis.

vation, the unchanged and deteriorated ones, however,
keep their initial values. Thus, there are remarkable
relations between the behaviour of plasma ammonia in
patients with CAH and their prognosis.
Already in CPH plasma ammonia is slightly increased
parallel to the inflammatory activity. Chronic infections
like in this case prostatitis cause an increase of serum
transaminases as well as of plasma ammonia.
An eight years follow-up control of a patient with HBsAg
positive CAH IIb is listed on fig. 2. After the discovery
and successful treatment of an open pulmonary tuberculo-
sis, a complete healing was obtained which is already
mentioned elsewhere. Parallel to the recession of
inflammatory activity, hyperammonemia decreases already
into normal before normalizing of the serum transaminases.
Finally one case of CAH which deteriorated permanently
during a long-term treatment with D-penicillamin.

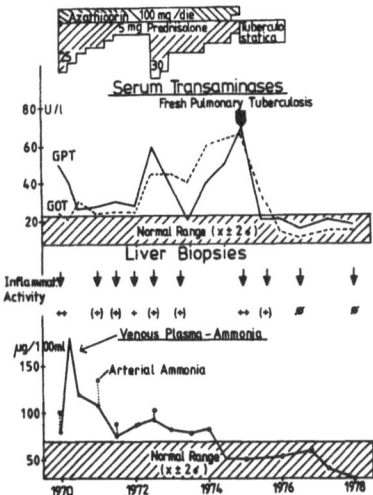

Fig. 2: Follow-up study of arterial and venous plasma
        ammonia in completely cured chronic active
        hepatitis.

This patient was controlled clinically, laparoscopically,
and bioptically over ten years. Parallel to the decrease
of his quick-value the plasma ammonia increased when a
severe portal hypertension developed. After all he died
in hepatic coma due to a severe necrotic exacerbation
(fig. 3).

How are the considerable disorders of the detoxification
capacity of the liver to be explained, regarding ammonia
and free phenols in CAH?

K. MAIER [4] called already in 1978 the attention of the
diminished activity of enzymes of the urea-cycle of the
liver in patients with CAH and enlarged his observations
in 1984. However, our patients had BUN-values in the
lower normal and the urea-excretion in 24 hrs urine with
a standard diet was only slightly diminished. Of course,
these methods are not as specific as the determination of
the enzyme activity in liver tissue.

We already mentioned, that free phenols are detoxified
by coupling on sulphuric acid and glucuronic acid. That

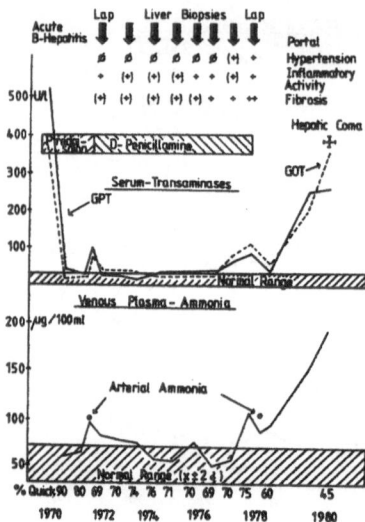

Fig. 3: Follow-up study of hyperammonemia in deteriorated chronic active hepatitis.

is the reason why the glucuronic acid level of the serum and urine is rather elevated in chronic hepatitis than in healthy adults, as former studies demonstrated[2].
In summary it is to be stated that patients with laparoscopically and histologically proven CAH have a distinctly decreased detoxification capacity of the liver. As well the urea synthesis in the liver as the coupling of phenols on glucuronic acid and sulphuric acid are diminished. That explains the significant increase of plasma ammonia and free phenols. This increase parallels to the inflammatory activity of the liver and the stage of cirrhotic transformation. The initially increased values of ammonia and phenols normalize in complete healing or defective healing. Lactulose and NH_3-reducing amino acids cause a decrease of the increased values of ammonia and phenols in CAH (5). The considerable psychical complaints like diminished mental capacity, depressions and tendency to aggressions are favorably influenced by this treatment. It seems to be important to pay more attention to the decreased detoxification capa-

city of the liver in CAH which, up to now, were too
little examined.

References

1. Wildhirt, E. (1969). Die Klinik der chronischen Hepatitis und ihre Differentialdiagnose. Dtsch.med.J.20.
   Jg., 492-496

2. Müting, D., Reikowski, H., Schmid, I. (1969). Eiweiß-
   stoffwechsel und Entgiftungsfunktion bei chronischer
   Hepatitis. Modern Gastroenterology, F.K. Schattauer-
   Verlag, Stuttgart

3. Müting, D., Winter, G., Fischer, R. et al. (1982). Is
   chronic active hepatitis curable? The Lancet, April
   17, 905-906

4. Maier, K.P., Talke, H., Gerok,W. (1978). Harnstoff-
   zyklusenzyme und Harnstoffsynthese bei chronischen
   Lebererkrankungen. In: Wewalka, F., Dragosics, B.:
   Aminosäuren, Ammoniak und hepatische Enzephalopathie.
   Fischer, Stuttgart, 33

5. Müting, D., Reikowski, J., Rosskopf, U. (1980).
   Bifidum-Milch und Laktulose in der Therapie chronischer
   Leberkrankheiten. Med.Welt 31, 22, 857-860

Reprints to:

Prof. Dr. D. Müting
Department Innere Medizin - Gastroenterologie
HEINZ KALK-Klinik

D - 8730 Bad Kissingen

10

Prognosis of Chronic Active Hepatitis: 10 years Follow-up Study in 144 Patients

D. MÜTING[1], G. WINTER[2], J.F. KALK[1] and R. FISCHER[1]

[1]Heinz Kalk-Klinik, Bad Kissingen
[2]Leopoldina hospital, Schweinfurt, F.R.G.

Zusammenfassung

144 Patienten mit einer leberbioptisch gesicherten chronisch-aktiven Hepatitis (CAH) wurden durchschnittlich 10 Jahre lang klinisch und ambulant kontrolliert. Von ihnen heilten 35 (24,3 %) völlig aus. Bei 27 (18,9 %) kam es zu einer Defektheilung in eine völlig inaktive Leberzirrhose, 20,8 % wurden gebessert, 13,9 % blieben unverändert, während sich 22,2 % deutlich verschlechterten. Bestimmend für die Prognose waren Ausmaß der entzündlichen Aktivität sowie HBsAg und HBeAg-Persistenz.
Von der Gruppe der 32 verschlechterten Patienten waren zwei Drittel HBs- und HBe-positiv, bei 6 entwickelte sich ein primäres Leberzellkarzinom. 66 % der mit Prednisolon behandelten Patienten klagten über erhebliche Nebenwirkungen (chronische Infekte, Magenerosionen und -ulcera, Glaukom, Katarakt), dagegen nur 11 % der Imurek-Patienten. Sowohl durch immunsuppressive Behandlung als auch durch eine Basistherapie mit Lactulose und ammoniaksenkenden Aminosäuren war in etwa gleichem Umfang eine völlige Ausheilung bzw. Besserung der CAH möglich, wenn sie lange genug durchgeführt wurde.

In the course of the past 20 years 650 patients in total
with chronic active hepatitis (CAH) were treated in the
HEINZ KALK-Clinic, Bad Kissingen, West Germany.
144 of them were controlled indoor and outdoor over 10
years on an average. The diagnosis was performed in all
cases by laparoscopy and liver biopsy. Each patient had
2 laparoscopies and 5 to 6 liver biopsies on an average.

We owe the morphology of the biopsies to Professor Wepler
and Professor Klinge of the Pathological Institute of the
Municipal Hospital Kassel. The results of these retrospective studies were as follows[1]. 35 of 144 patients
are completely cured. 27 were defectively cured i.e.
completely inactive liver cirrhosis. 30 were improved,
which means 64 % showed a clear therapeutical success.
20 patients remained unchanged. In 32 patients the
pathological picture deteriorated distinctly, pointing
to an active posthepatitic liver cirrhosis (fig. 1).
Which factors favoured the relatively good results of
this retrospective long-term study?
First it has to be mentioned that we treated with few
exceptions only patients without cirrhotic transformation and most of all without portal hypertension. Here-
with we are in contrary to the results of most of the

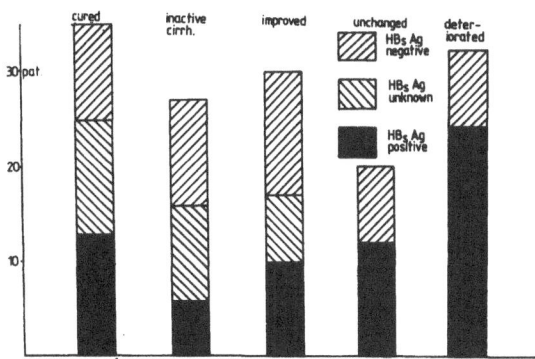

Fig. 1: Importance of HBsAg-persistence for the prognosis
         of chronic-active hepatitis after 10-years
         treatment (n = 144)

Anglosaxon controlled double blind studies of the so-
called "chronic active hepatitis". As success they
compared only the survival time of patients treated with
prednisolone alone, azathioprin alone or the combination
of both substances with a placebo-group [2,3,4,5]. In
these 6 studies 20 - 40 % of deaths appeared already in
the placebo-group due to oesophageal variceal hemorrhages
or hepatic coma, signs of severe portal hypertension
(pH). This high percentage of ph in the Anglosaxon
patients is due to not performing laparoscopies or at
least regular gastroscopies in order to exclude oesophageal varices, but only needle puncture. Beside of the
not existing ph 2 more factors play an important role of
the prognosis of our 144 patients with CAH: HBsAg-persistence and the severity of inflammatory activity of
the liver.

Fig. 1 shows the percentage of HBsAg-persistence in 5
collectives of our 144 patients with CAH. While only
20-30 % of the cured or improved patients were HBsAg
positive, the deteriorated ones had a rate of 80 %. As
we started our examinations long before 1973, when the
determination of Australia-Antigen was introduced, we
also are in possession of a smaller collective of
patients with CAH where these analyses were not yet
possible.

Fig. 2 indicates the severity of inflammatory activity
of the liver in our 144 patients. As known, CAH is
devided in type IIa with slight to moderate activity and
type IIb with high inflammatory activity. In this distribution the percentage of both types regarding the cured
and improved cases is about equal. In the unchanged and
especially the deteriorated patients type IIb with high
inflammatory activity has the major part.

Beside of the starting conditions like HBsAg-persistence
and inflammatory activity also the duration of the
immunosuppressive therapy is important for the prognosis.
In fig. 3 our 144 patients are devided according to their

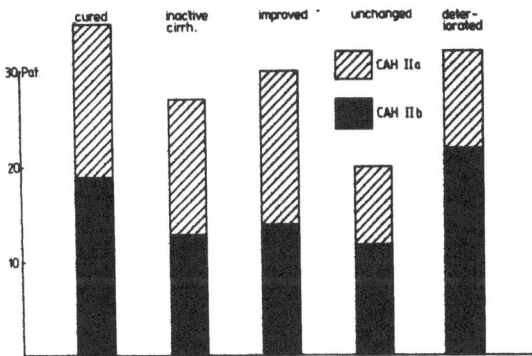

Fig. 2: Importance of inflammatory activity for the
prognosis of chronic-active hepatitis after
10-years treatment (n≐144)

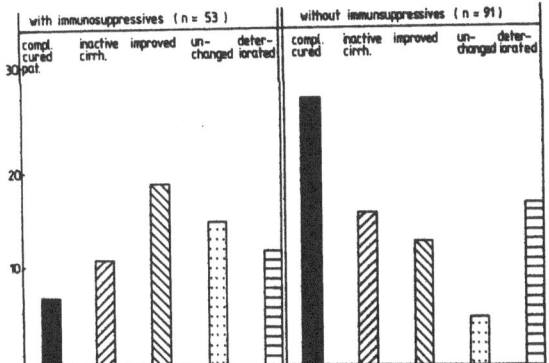

Fig. 3: 10-years treatment of chronic-active hepatitis
(n=144) with and without immunosuppressive
substances

therapy in 2 groups such as on the left with immunosuppressives (53) and on the right without those (91).
It is a remarkable fact that the group without immunosuppressives shows four times more healings than after
treatment with prednisolone-azathioprin. Of course, one
may argue that presumably the HBsAg-persistence and
inflammatory activity were primarily less in this group
and therefore immunosuppressives were not needed. The
percentage of CAH IIa was really higher in the group
without immunosuppressives because according to the usual
rules only CAH IIb is an indication for a long-term
treatment with immunosuppressives.

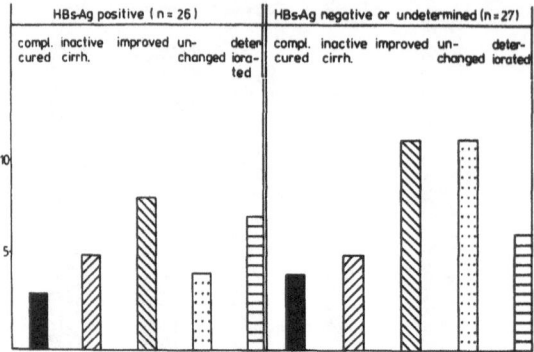

Fig. 4: Results of a 10-years treatment of chronic-active hepatitis with immunosuppressive substances (n=53)

The HBsAg-persistence is another matter of fact. We researched again for the appearance of HBsAg in 53 patients who received immunosuppressives (fig. 4). The therapeutical success in both groups concerning healing and defective healing turned out to be nearly equal. Hence, there is no reason to fall into therapeutical nihilism when CAH IIb with HBsAg-persistence is present, as SCHALM (6) declared sharply in last time. However, it is absolutely necessary to reduce the maintenance dose of prednisolone to a minimum of 7.5 to 12.5 mg per day in order to avoid dangerous side effects.

These are summarized on table 1. For prednisolone they amount to 66 %, for azathioprin (75 mg/die on an average) to 12 % only. Side effects due to more than 15 mg%/die of prednisolone are: chronic pancreatitis, osteoporosis, psychosis and more and more cataract and glaucoma. Doses under 15 mg cause a diminished resistence against acute and chronic infections. The severest complication in a long-term treatment of CAH should not be concealed, the primary liver cell carcinoma.

Out of 30 deteriorated patients 24 were HBs- and HBeAg positive. 8 patients of them developed a primary liver cell carcinoma, thus one third. Since we performed yearly controls by ultrasound, laparoscopy and computer

Table 1: Side effects of long-term treatment with
immunosuppressives in CAH

A. Prednisolone (44 of 67 pat.= 66 %)		B. Azathioprin (4 of 32 pat.= 12 %)	
1. steroid diabetes	11	1. leucopenia	3
2. chronic infections	11	2. sexual insufficiency	1
3. chronic pancreatitis	5		
4. acute psychosis	5		
5. ulcus duodeni	4		
6. hypokaliemia	2		
7. cataracta	2		
8. steroid acne	2		
9. glaucoma	1		

tomography in patients with a process of disease for more than 5 years, we found 4 more cases of primary liver cell carcinoma. One of them had a successful liver resection, another one had a liver transplant.

In the short disposable time only the most important problems were touched which seem to be significant for the prognosis of CAH.

In summary it has to be mentioned that the exclusion of portal hypertension, if possible of complete liver cirrhosis, slight inflammatory activity and negative HBsAg facilitates essentially the healing. Fortunately, a healing of CAH IIa with HBsAg persistence is possible if the long-term treatment with prednisolone and azathioprin is performed in a most low maintenance dose (7).

References

1. Müting, D., Winter, G., Fischer, R., Kruck, P., Kalk, H. (1982). Is chronic active hepatitis curable? The Lancet, april 17

2. Cook, G.C., Mulligan, R., Sherlock, S. (1971). Controlled prospective tial of corticoid therapy in active chronic hepatitis. Quart.J.Med.40, 159

3. Mackay, I.R. (1972). The prognosis of chronic hepatitis. Am. Int. Med. 77, 649
4. Murray-Lyon, I. (1973). Controlled trial of prednisolone and azathioprine in active chronic hepatitis.
   The Lancet I, 735 - 737
5. Soloway, R.D., Summerskill, W.H.J., Bagenstoss, A.H.
   et al. (1972). Clinical, biochemical and histological
   remission of severe chronic active liver disease: a
   controlled study of treatment and early diagnosis.
   Gastroenterology 63, 820 - 833
6. Schalm, S.W. (1981). Soll die chronisch aktive Virushepatitis medikamentös behandelt werden oder nicht?
   Internist 22, 717-720
7. Müting, D., Winter, G., Fischer, R. and Kalk, J.F.
   (1984). Treatment of chronic active hepatitis -
   present state. Hepato-Gastroenterology No.1, Vol.31,
   17 - 23

Reprints to:

Prof. Dr. D. Müting
Department Innere Medizin - Gastroenterologie
HEINZ KALK-Klinik

D - 8730 Bad Kissingen

11

Prognosis of Patients with Liver Cirrhosis and History of Variceal Bleeding after Spleno-renal and Mesocaval Shunt using Two Different Selection Criteria for Shunt Operation

K.-J. PAQUET, P. KOUSSOURIS and H.-J. BIERSACK

Department of Surgery, Heinz Kalk-Klinik, Bad Kissingen and Institute of Nuclear Medicine, University of Bonn, W. Germany

Zusammenfassung

Vom 01.01.75 - 01.01.83 wurden die Selektionskriterien Lebervolumen, Pfortaderhochdruckströmung, Ausschluß einer Aktivität der Leberzirrhose und einer Stenose im arteriellen Zuflußgebiet der Leber in einer prospektiven Untersuchung für die Auswahl von 102 Patienten für eine elektive und selektive bzw. semi-selektive Shuntoperation überprüft. Dieses Patientenkollektiv (Gruppe II) wurde einer Gruppe I von 101 Patienten gegenübergestellt, die vom 01.01.59 - 01.01.75 einer elektiven, selektiven und semi-selektiven Shuntoperation zugeführt worden waren, wobei man zur Auswahl konventionelle Kriterien nach CHILD verwandt hatte. Beide Patientenkollektive waren in wesentlichen Kriterien vergleichbar mit Ausnahme des Verhältnisses von alkohol-toxischer zu anderen Formen der Zirrhose. Der Vergleich beider Kollektive ergab eine statistisch hochsignifikante Verbesserung der Früh- und Spätergebnisse im zweiten Behandlungszeitraum. Die angewandten Selektionskriterien haben somit ihre Bewährungsprobe bestanden; ohne ihre Berücksichtigung sollte kein Patient mehr einer elektiven Shuntoperation zugeführt werden.

Liver insufficiency in cirrhotic patients with portal
hypertension after a shunt operation is mainly caused by
the decrease of the already diminished portal blood
supply to the liver. This is especially true when the
arterial supply does not increase as may be the case
after total deviation of the portal blood to the vena
cava inferior following a termino-lateral porto-caval
anastomosis. - The aims of the surgical efforts during
the last 15 years therefore consisted of developping
surgical methods, which are able to preserve partially
or totally the liver perfusion (2,7). Besides this surgical progress efforts were made to find out physical and
hemodynamic criteria, which can facilitate the prediction
of operative risks and long-term prognosis of shunt
operations.

There is a close and highly significant correlation between liver volume and oxygen consumption of the liver.
In case of enlargement or diminution of the volume of a
cirrhotic liver there is an increase of oxygen consumption without a relative functional effect. Whether hepatic tissue is sufficiently perfused after a shunt operation depends on the relation between liver volume and
total liver perfusion, i.e. the perfusion index. These
data must be taken into consideration for selection of
patients for a shunt operation. The liver should not be
less than 1000 ml and not more than 2500 ml in volume
(3,6). As non-invasive and clinical relevant nuclear
method for the pre- and postoperative determination of
total liver and portal perfusion the sequential hepato-
spleno-scintigraphy with 99m-Tc-Pertechnate and Radio-
colloid-clearance with 99m-Tc-Sulfurcolloid have been
developped by us (1,5,6). The quantitative sequential
perfusion-scintigraphy is moreover a proper method for.
the determination of the relation between arterial and
portal perfusion of the liver. These two criteria are
completed by laparoscopy in combination with biopsy to
exclude activity and progress of the liver process (4)

Table 1:   Selection criteria for elective shunts in liver
           cirrhosis after variceal hemorrhage

---

1. Determination of liver volume by sonography
   (limits: between 1000 and 2500 ml) -
   controlled by laparoscopy

2. Determination of portal perfusion by sequential
   scintigraphy (at least 15 %) -
   controlled by selective angiography

3. Laparoscopy and biopsy

4. Selective lieno-, hepatico-, mesentericography and
   indirect lieno-, mesenterico-portography (arterial
   hepatic blood supply-lumen and length of the
   shunted vein)

---

and selective visceral angiography to exclude a stenosis
of the arterial supply to the liver (Tab. 1).
The value of the above mentioned methods for the estimation of the early and long-term results after selective
or semi-selective shunt operations was tested for a
period of 8 years. The results will be referred to the
long-term results of a similar collective of patients
which have been previously operated upon using conventional criteria (2) (Tab. 2).

Tab. 2:   Indications for elective shunt operation in
          liver cirrhosis after variceal hemorrhage
          (01.01.69 - 01.01.75

---

1. Compensated liver function (CHILD and PAQUET
   criterial);

2. biochemical exclusion of an activity of the liver
   process;

3. exclusion of preoperative hepatoportal encephalopathy;

4. no high morbidity of other diseases;

5. age up to 65 years.

Material and methods

101 patients with liver cirrhosis and a history of one or
more bleedings from esophageal varices were operated upon
with a spleno-renal anastomosis after LINTON or WARREN in
the period from January 1st, 1969, to January 1st, 1975
and have been followed up for at least 8 years (Tab. 3).

Table 3: Confrontation of shunt types of group I
         (performed from January 1st, 1969, to January
         1st, 1975) and group II (performed from January
         1st, 1975, to January 1st, 1983) in the
         Department of Surgery, University of Bonn, and
         Heinz Kalk-Clinic, Bad Kissingen, West Germany

Group I		Group II	
Type	Number	Type	Number
Conventional spleno-renal shunt (LINTON)	84	Conventional spleno-renal shunt (LINTON)	28
Distal splenorenal shunt (WARREN)	17	Distal splenorenal shunt (WARREN)	8
		Mesocaval inter-position shunt (DRAPANAS)	66
	101		102

The underlying disease of this group I was a liver cirrhosis in 93 %. The criteria for the selection of this
group of patients for an elective shunt operation are
described in Tab. 2. It must be emphasized that from this
statistical analysis patients with porto-caval anastomosis have been excluded. Since January 1st, 1975 we do not
carry out this operation anymore because of a high rate
of postoperative mortality (14 %), encephalopathy (25 %)
and a progressive deterioration of liver function for
about 50 % in the first 3 postoperative years.

This collective of patients (group I) is compared to
102 patients with liver cirrhosis (95 %) and a history of
one or more bleedings from esophageal varices which were

operated upon from 01.01.75 - 01.01.83 electively
(group II). Since 01.01.75 the criteria listed up in
Tab. 1 had to be fulfilled to be allowed to carry out an
elective shunt operation. The different types of shunts
in both groups are compared in Tab. 3. Both groups are
comparable to each other (Tab. 4) with exception of the
relation of the alcoholic type of cirrhosis to other
types.

Table 4: Comparison of clinical features in group I and
         group II

	Group I (n=101)	Group II (n=102)
Age (years)	52	50
Sex	71 M/30 F	68 M/34 F
Cirrhosis	93 %	94 %
Results of liver biopsy Ratio of alcoholic to non-alcoholic cirrhosis	1,9 : 1,0	2,4 : 1,0
CHILD-classification	A (70 %) B (30 %)	A (72 %) B (28 %)
Frequency of variceal hemorrhage	2	2
Number of blood transfusion	6	7

Results

The examinations done in every patient for the diagnosis
of encephalopathy have been carried out very extensively
and with high accuracy. The early and long-term results
are compared in Fig. 1.

There is no doubt that the results in the second period
are significantly better. Thus it is no longer justified
today to perform an elective shunt operation without
using these selection criteria preoperatively.

Abstract
An selection criteria for an elective shunt operation
from January 1st, 1975 to January 1st, 1983 patients with

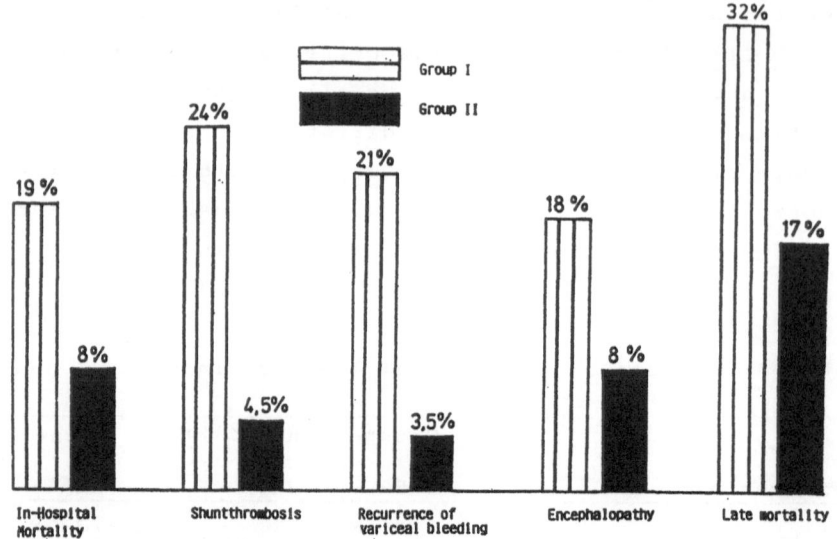

Figure 1

liver cirrhosis after variceal hemorrhage liver volume,
portal perfusion and no activity supply of the liver have
been tested in a prospective evaluation of 102 shunt
operations. This group II was compared to group I of
101 patients operated upon from 01.01.69 - 01.01.85 using
conventional selection criteria during the bleeding free
intervall. Porto-caval anastomoses of group I were
excluded of the statistical analysis. The two groups were
comparable in all essential criteria with exception of
the ratio of the alcoholic type to other types of cirrhosis. During the second period early and long-term
results were significantly better. Therefore these selection criteria have proven a high accuracy and reliability
for the selection of patients for elective, selective and
semi-selective shunt operations.

References

1. Biersack, H.J., Thelen, M., Paquet, K.-J., Knopp, R.,
   Schmidt, R., Winkler, C. (1977). Die sequentielle
   Hepato-spleno-Szintigraphie zur quantitativen Beurteilung der Leberdurchblutung. Fortschr. Röntgenstr.
   126,   47

2. Child, C.G. (1964). III The liver and portal hypertension. W.B. Saunders, Philadelphia

3. Koischwitz, D. (1979). Sonographische Lebervolumenbestimmung: Problematik, Methodik und praktische Bedeutung der Quantifizierung des Lebervolumens. Fortschr. Röntgenstr. 131, 243

4. Mikkelsen, W.P., Torrill, F.L., Kern, W.H. (1968). Acute hyaline necrosis of the liver: a surgical trap. Am.J. Surg. 116, 266

5. Paquet, K.-J., Thelen, M., Koischwitz, G. Biersack,H.J. (1979). Ein neues therapeutisches Konzept für die Auswahl von Leberzirrhotikern mit rezidivierender Ösophagusvarizenblutung für den elektiven Shunt. Chirurg, 50, 313

6. Paquet, K.-J., Janson, R., Biersack, H.J. (1982). Spätergebnisse nach splenorenalem und mesokavalem Shunt beim Leberzirrhotiker. Vergleich zweier verschiedener Selektionskriterien. Arch.Klin.Chir., 358, 475

7. Price, J.B.jr., Voorhees, A.B.jr. Britton, R.C. (1967) Operative hemodynamics in portal hypertension. Arch. Surg., 95, 843

Reprints to:

Prof. Dr. med. K.-J. Paquet
Department für Chirurgie - Gefäßchirurgie
HEINZ KALK-Klinik

D - 8730 Bad Kissingen

12
On the Prognosis of Liver Cirrhosis

M. BURGHARDT, A. HENZE, U. RUSSMANN, J. LOBERS, E. SCHMIDT and F.W. SCHMIDT

Abt. Gastroenterologie und Hepatologie, Zentrum Innere Medizin und Dermatologie, Medizinische Hochschule, Hannover, F.R.G.

Zusammenfassung

Mit dem Ziel anhand von 10 klinischen, 12 klinisch-
chemischen und allen verfügbaren morphologischen Befunden
die Prognose für den einzelnen Patienten mit Lebercirrhose zu ermitteln, wurden 1 145 Kranken-Akten retro-
spektiv untersucht und fehlende Befunde von auswärts
eingeholt. Die Auswertung, der nach Aetiologie gruppier-
ten und nach dem Todesdatum synchronisierten Krankheits-
verläufe der 658 bereits verstorbenen Patienten brachte
als erstes Ergebnis Klarheit über die Unzulänglichkeit
statistischer Vergleiche von Gruppendaten für eine indi-
viduelle Prognostik und die Notwendigkeit einer zugleich
differenzierten und synoptischen Betrachtung, wobei
neben.dem Ausmaß die Geschwindigkeit der pathologischen
Veränderungen wahrscheinlich erhebliche Bedeutung zukommt.

The increasing success of aggressive forms of treatment -
like the replacement of a cirrhotic liver by a liver
graft - compels the attending physician to determine the
right point of time for this measure; with other words:
he must decide, how good or how bad the prognosis of his
individual patient is at any given time.

According to the literature, the average 5-years survival rate of patients with cirrhosis of the liver has been enlarged from 18 % between 1942 - 1974 up to 50 % or even 72 % in patients without ascites, in recent years (1, 2, 3, 4). The prolongation of life was only partly due to better therapy, but mostly to better diagnostics. This has been demonstrated by WILDHIRT and ORTMANS (5), who by frequent serial examinations of their patients with chronic hepatitis detected the cirrhotic transformation very early and, starting their calculations from this point, report on survival rates of 74 % even after 15 years.

Besides the stage, when recognized, the severity of the liver damage is the decisive prognostic factor: Patients in stage C after Child have a 3 - 6 times lesser chance to survive 5 years than patients in stage A after Child (6).

However, the reported data on survival of cirrhotics depend on the composition of the collectives and are therefore of little value for the appraisal of the future in individual patients. For years, this notion has stimulated the search for objective, easily available clinical signs or repeatable laboratory investigations, which alone or combined, like e.g. the Child Index (7) or the CCLI (8) would serve to assess prognosis in the individual case.

The life expectancy of a patient with liver cirrhosis can be limited due to a variety of permanent threats or un-expected deleterious events. Thus, the problem of indivi-dual prognostication is so multifacetted that it can only be solved by modern computing devices, if at all.

The aim of our retrospective study was to find patterns of selected parameters for the early recognition, if, when and how much an individual patient is in jeopardy by imminent liver failure, massive bleeding or the sequelae of his weakened immune reactions and metabolic capacities.

Material and Methods

The files of 1,145 patients, who were treated under the diagnosis "Cirrhosis of the Liver" at the Hannover School of Medicine were investigated. By documentation of etiology and begin of the liver disease, of the assessment of diagnosis, of therapy, complications, survival, causes of death and autoptic findings, and, particularly, by listing 10 clinical and 12 laboratory signs and the morphological examinations throughout the course, the individual course of the disease was delineated.

Additional data were obtained from 535 familiy doctors and senior physicians of other hospitals and more than 50 social institutions and insurances (With 80 % replies the cooperation was outstanding, which we gratefully acknowledge).

From the multitude of clinical and laboratory data two patterns per annum were selected at the date of the highest and of the lowest ASAT activity in serum, reflecting the presence or absence of acute exacerbations and the general type of the course.

Results and Discussion

Table 1 shows that of the 1,145 patients 658 are already deceased. It shows that with respect to the distribution of age, sex and the etiology of cirrhosis the group of the deceased is virtually identical to the total collective. Therefore, we have considered the former representative for the total population of patients with liver cirrhosis attending to our hospital. Only this group has been evaluated further up to now.

Table 2 shows the distribution of age and sex, and the survival times after the diagnosis of cirrhosis in the four main etiological subgroups, which comprise hearly

Table 1 :

PATIENTS	Total (%)		Deceased (%)	
Number	1,145	(100)	658	(57)
Male	759	(66)	432	(66)
Female	386	(34)	226	(34)
Age (years)	n	(%)	n	(%)
below 20	2	(0.2)	1	(0.2)
20 - 29	41	(3.6)	20	(3.1)
30 - 39	144	(12.6)	63	(9.7)
40 - 49	269	(23.5)	146	(22.5)
50 - 59	329	(28.7)	185	(28.5)
60 - 69	221	(19.3)	141	(21.7)
70 - 79	121	(10.6)	79	(12.2)
80 - 89	16	(1.4)	12	(1.8)
above 90	2	(0.2)	2	(0.3)
Etiology of cirrhosis	n	(%)	n	(%)
Viral hepatitis B	110	(9.6)	67	(10.2)
Viral hepatitis NANB	18	(1.6)	9	(1.4)
Viral hepatitis unspecified	135	(11.8)	78	(11.8)
Alcohol toxic	596	(52.1)	330	(50.2)
Primary biliary	33	(2.9)	20	(3.0)
Secondary biliary	12	(1.1)	6	(0.9)
Hemochromatosis	7	(0.6)	3	(0.5)
Cryptogenetic	234	(20.4)	145	(22.0)

99 % of all patients. The mean survival time is rather
short in all four groups, but the range is very wide.

After synchronization of the individual courses back-
wards from the date of death, 6 laboratory parameters
were chosen for a first overall attempt to select
suitable candidates for prognostic indices. Three of
them are traditionally components of prognostic

Table 2 : Different etiology of cirrhosis: sex - age -
          survival rates

Etiology	male/female % %	Age at diagnosis Mean (range) years	Survival rates Mean (range) years
Hepatitic (23.4 %)	66 34	54.7 (20 - 70)	3.4 (1 - 29)
Toxic (50.2 %)	74 26	50.8 (20 - 90)	2.5 (1 - 19)
Cryptogen. (22.0 %)	58 42	63.2 (20 - 80)	4.1 (1 - 32)
PBC (3.0 %)	10 90	51.0 (20 - 60)	4.5 (1 - 12)

indices : Prothrombin time, albumin and bilirubin.
The other three have proven us useful for the
assessment of individual progression :   CHE, ALAT
and GGT.

Fig. 1 a-c shows the course of the two medians (at
highest and lowest ASAT activity of the year) of the six
parameters during the 5 years before death. The courses
of hepatitic, toxic and cryptogenetic cirrhoses are
considered separately. The prothrombin time decreases in
two steps, most pronounced in the hepatitic type, least
in the toxic one. In contrast, the rise of the bilirubin
is most marked in toxic cirrhosis and begins 1 - 2 years
earlier than the final drop of GGT. Cholinesterase levels
fall more gradually; slower and faster phases seem to
exist, though, again best visible in the toxic type. It
is evident that - in our population - albumin and ALAT
as such cannot considered to be candidates for a prognostic index, although the diminuition of the latter leads
to the increase of the DRQ, which is prognostically
rather reliable (9), and contributes significantly to the
detection of primary hepatocellular carcinoma (10).

The four remaining parameters have been for their
suitability in individual prediction, again in the three
big etiological groups as wholes. In Fig. 2 a and b the

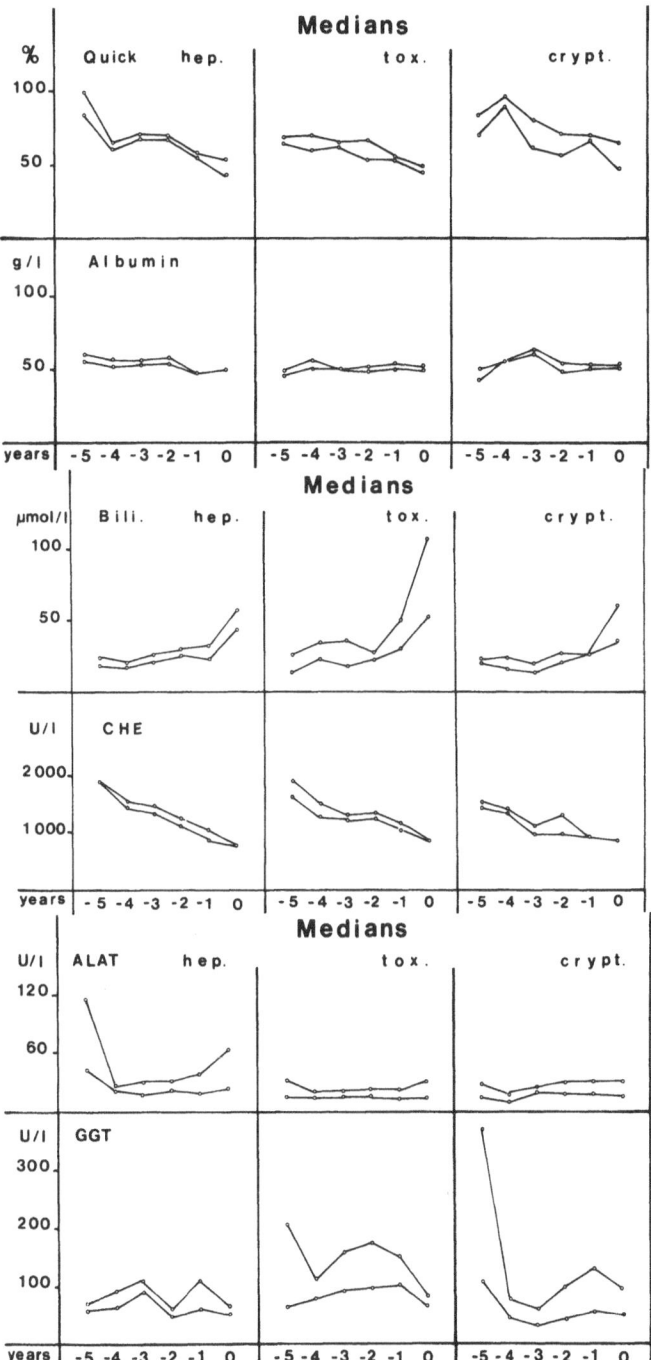

Fig. 1: Medians of 6 parameters, biennual at the dates of
the highest and the lowest ASAT activity in serum
of the year.
Abscissa: 0 = year of death

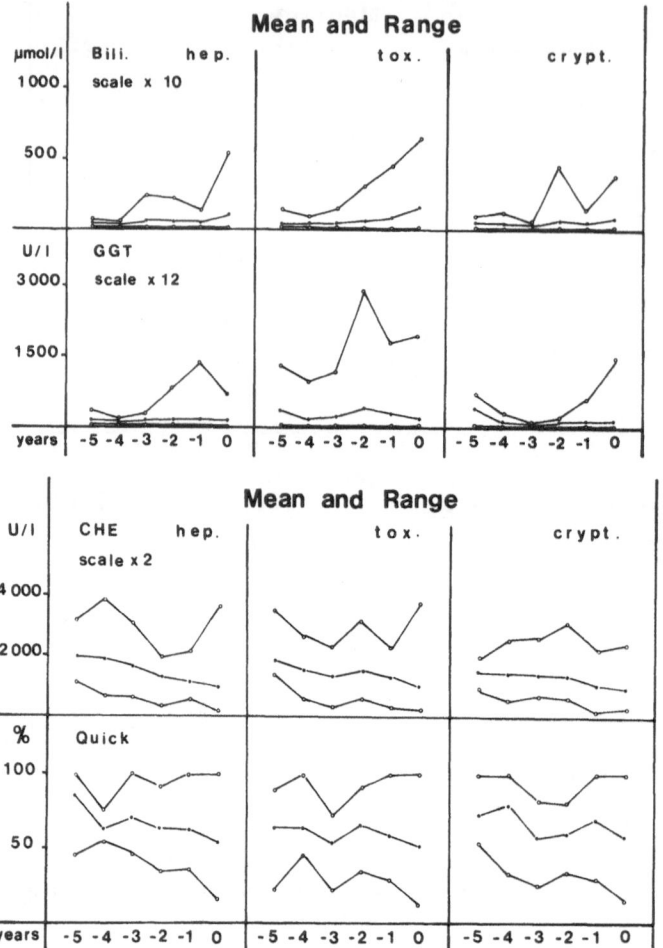

Fig. 2: Mean values and ranges of 4 parameters, biennual
at the dates of the highest and the lowest ASAT
activity in serum of the year.
Abscissa: 0 = year of death

5-years prefinal courses of the mean values and of the
upper and lower limits of the ranges are demonstrated.

The result is disappointing, as could be expected:
Although the mean and the extreme values of bilirubin
rise, normal bilirubin concentrations can be found until
death. The prefinal decrease of GGT is only reproduced by
its mean activity in toxic cirrhosis, whereas the general
tendency of the upper limit values is to rise during the

last years, possibly as a sign of unrecognized liver cancer. Prothrombin time and CHE show a better correlation between mean and lowest, most pathological values during the last years. However, the upper limit values lie always or particularly prefinally within the reference range. If this is due to therapeutical substitution, e.g. after bleeding, these tests become, of course, useless for prognostication.

Conclusions

From our very preliminary results, the only conclusion can be that prognostic indices based on statistical evaluation only are of little use for the individual patient. If statistical patterns shall be established, which can be used as basis for therapeutical decisions, a multifacetted approach is necessary. It has to begin with the classification of the causes of death in the different stages of liver cirrhosis of various types, and may end up with the description of the extent and the velocity of changes in the course of the disease.

Abbreviations

ALAT   Alanin aminotransferase (E.C. 2.6.1.2)

ASAT   Aspartate aminotransferase (E.C. 2.6.1.1)

CCLI   Combined Clinical and Laboratory Index

CHE   Cholinesterase (E.C. 3.1.1.8)

GGT   Gamma-glutamyl-transferase (E.C. 2.3.2.2)

DRQ   DeRitis ratio: ASAT / ALAT

References

1) Ratnoff, O.D., Patek,A.J.(1942).Medicine 21, 207

2) Creutzfeld, W., Beck, K. (1966). Dtsch.med.Wschr. 91, 682

3) Eisenburg, J.(1984). Lebensversicherungsmedizin 6, 129

4) Pagliaro, L., D'Amico, G., Morabito, A., Marubini,E., Pasta,L., Caltagirone, M., Traina,M. (1983). Congress of the European Association for the Study of the Liver.

5) Ortmans,H., Wildhirt,E. (1975). Dtsch.med.Wschr.<u>100</u>,
   812

6) Marosi, L., Ferenci,P., Dragosics, B., Kiss, F.,
   Pollack C.H., Minar, E. (1983). Schweiz.med.Wschr.
   <u>113</u>, 1586

7) Child, C.G., Turcott, J.G. (1964). In: C.G. Child,
   The liver and portal hypertension. W.B.Saunders Co.
   Philadelphia, p. 50

8) Rink, C.H.R., Otto, L. (1982).Dt.Gesundh.Wesen <u>37</u>,540

9) Schmidt, E. (1974). In: L. Wannagat, Chronische
   Hepatitis - Zirrhosen. Thieme Stuttgart, p.85

10) Aramaki,T., Hanyuda, Y., Akaike, M., Nagasava, K.,
   Okumura, H., Hayashi, C. (1984). Congress of the
   International Association for the Study of the Liver.

Reprints to:

Prof. Dr.F.W. Schmidt
Abt. Gastroenterologie u. Hepatologie
Medizinische Hochschule Hannover
Konstanty Gutschow Str. 8

D - 3000 Hannover 61

Portal Circulation

13
Effect of Nitroglycerin on Portal Hypertension

G.H. BÜTZOW, E. WINDLER, H. RAMMOSER and F. LEMPP

Medizinische Kernklinik und Poliklinik, Universitäts – Krankenhaus Eppendorf, Hamburg

Zusammenfassung

Bei bisher 15 Patienten mit dekompensierter Leberzirrhose überwiegend alkoholischer Genese und mit Pfortaderhochdruck wurde der Effekt von 0,8 mg Glyceroltrinitrat auf den indirekten Pfortaderdruck (geblockter minus freier Lebervenenddruck, WHVP-FHVP) über 30 Minuten gemessen. Vorher und nachher wurde das Herzzeitvolumen mittels Thermodilutionsmethode, der arterielle Blutdruck und die Herzfrequenz registriert. Nach 4 Wochen wurden die gleichen Messungen bei 5 Patienten unter 2 x 100 mg Metoprolol und bei 5 unbehandelten Kontrollpersonen wiederholt.

Die orale Nitroglyzeringabe führte zu einer Drucksenkung (WHVP-FHVP) von x = 21,9 $\pm$ 6,0 auf 17,2 $\pm$ 6,2 mm Hg (p 0,012). Lediglich bei einem Patienten wurde keine Drucksenkung beobachtet. Das Herzzeitvolumen sank von $\bar{x}$ = 7,81 $\pm$ 1,08 auf 6,72 $\pm$ 0,78 l/min (p 0,0025) ab. Der systolische arterielle Blutdruck fiel von $\bar{x}$ = 136 $\pm$ 22 auf 123 $\pm$ 21 mmHg bei konstanter Herzfrequenz ($\bar{x}$ = 85 $\pm$ 15 vs. 80 $\pm$ 14). Unter ß-Rezeptorenblockern senkte Nitroglyzerin zusätzlich den bereits reduzierten Pfortaderdruck um durchschnittlich 4,8 mmHg (p 0,01).

Diese Ergebnisse zeigen, daß bei Patienten mit dekompensierter Leberzirrhose und portaler Hypertension durch

orale Nitroglyzeringabe akut eine Drucksenkung um durchschnittlich 20 % möglich ist. Offenbar kann Nitroglyzerin
eine durch ß-Rezeptorenblocker induzierte Drucksenkung
verstärken. Weitere Studien sind erforderlich, um den
klinischen Wert von Nitropräparaten in der Blutungsthera-
pie und Blutungsprophylaxe abschätzen zu können.

Introduction

The portal pressure depends on portal blood flow and
intra- und extrahepatic vascular resistance. Drugs lowering the portal pressure could act through both of these
factors.
So far, decrease of portal pressure has only been achieved by reduction of cardiac output or constriction of
splanchnic arterioles, i.e. by diminution of portal flow.
Nitroglycerin is reported to reduce cardiac output
through venous pooling, but also by decreasing the tonus
of hepatic venules. Thus, lowering of the intrahepatic
vascular resistance can be expected with this drug. There
are only few data on the effect of nitroglycerin in
portal hypertension. Therefore, we investigated the acute
effect of nitroglycerin in patients with portal hypertension and liver cirrhosis and the additive effect in
patients on ß - blockers.

Patients and Methods

15 patients with decompensated liver cirrhosis and portal
hypertension (12 men and 3 women) were investigated.
The etiology of liver cirrhosis was alcoholic in 11
cases, posthepatitic in 3 cases and unknown in one
patient. All but two patients had increased bilirubin
(0.7 - 16.8 mg/dl). Only one patient had no ascites. Four
patients had grade I, seven patients grade II and two
patients no hepatic encephalopathy, which was quantified
by means of the number-connection-test. All but two
patients had oesophageal varices verified by endoscopy,
the grade of which varied between grade I and grade IV

of a subjective scale. The gradient between free and wedged hepatic venous pressure was 21.9 + 6.0 mmHg (mean +
1 SD), range 15 - 39 mmHg. Initially in all patients a
four channel thermistor balloon catheter was placed in
the pulmonary artery and cardiac output was measured by
the thermodilution technique. Subsequently the catheter
was introduced into a hepatic vein and free and wedged
hepatic venous pressure were measured (FHVP, WHVP).
After sublingual application of 0.8 mg glyceroltrinitrate,
hepatic venous pressure was recorded in 5 minutes intervals for 30 minutes. After this half an hour period there
was a final measurement of the cardiac output.
Additionally pulse rate and arterial blood pressure were
registered before and after the catheterization procedure.
All patients, who gave their consent and who had no
contraindication, were randomized and underwent a treatment with a daily dose of 200 mg Metoprolol orally for
four weeks, or got no such therapy (control). After four
weeks the same catheterization procedure as above was
repeated. The entire investigation was completed in five
patients on ß-blockers and five controls. Differences
were evaluated by students t-test for paired observations.
A p of less than 0.05 was considered statistically
significant.

Results
In all but two of 20 investigations - among them 5
duplicate measurements in control patients - administration of nitroglycerin resulted in a decrease of the
hepatic venous pressure gradient (WHVP - FHVP)of at least
2 mmHg (range -2 to -19 mmHg). The mean decrease was
statistically highly significant (Table 1). As expected,
cardiac output decreased by about 1 l/min and the
systolic arterial blood pressure dropped slightly, but
statistically significant, while the pulse rate remained
unchanged. The effect of the four weeks course of ß -
blockers was similar to previous results (1), but did not

Table 1: Acute effect of 0.8 mg glycerolnitrate
sublingually.
Results including five repetitive
measurements in controls are given as
mean ± 1 SD.

	n	initial	Nitro	p
WHVP-FHVP (mmHg)	20	21.9 ± 6.0	17.2 ± 6.2	◄ 0.01
CO (1.min^{-1})	19	7.81 ± 1.08	6.72 ± 0.78	◄ 0.0025
BP (mmHg) syst.	20	136 ± 22	123 ± 21	◄ 0.025
diast.	20	79 ± 13	74 ± 12	n.s.
HR (min.$^{-1}$)	19	85 ± 15	83 ± 16	n.s.

Abbreviations: WHVP: wedged hepatic venous pressure.
FHVP: free hepatic venous pressure.
CO: cardiac output.
BP: blood pressure.
HR: heart rate.

reach statistical significance as the number of cases was
small and two patients did not respond to the drug
(Table 2). Administration of nitroglycerin during the
course of Metoprolol led in all investigated patients to
a further and statistically significant decrease of the
hepatic venous pressure gradient (range -1 to -7 mm Hg).
There was also a further decrease of the cardiac output,
while blood pressure and pulse rate were unaffected. In
none of the patients taking ß-blockers clinical or
laboratory findings deteriorated, especially there was no
worsening of encephalopathy as judged by number-connec-
tion-tests.

Discussion
The criteria for the selection of the investigated
patients were the presence of portal hypertension,
established diagnosis of liver cirrhosis, and at least
one sign of decompensation as icterus, ascites, or
encephalopathy. Although in two patients no oesophageal
varices could be demonstrated, the gradient between wed-

Table 2 : Acute effect of 0.8 mg glycerolnitrate with or without a four weeks course of 200 mg Metoprolol daily.

	n	HR (min^{-1})	WHVP-FHVP (mmHg) initial	WHVP-FHVP (mmHg) Nitro	p
initial	5	86 $\pm$ 9	22.2 $\pm$ 9.6	19.8 $\pm$ 10.9	▼ 0.1
after 4 weeks Metoprolol	5	67 $\pm$ 5	18.6 $\pm$ 6.4	13.8 $\pm$ 5.8	▼ 0.01
p	-	▼ 0.025	n.s.	-	

Abbrevations: WHVP: wedged hepatic venous pressure.

FHVP: free hepatic venous pressure.

HR: heart rate.

ged and free hepatic venous pressure of 15 mmHg or more
was in all patients markedly elevated (normal: up to
5 mmHg). With 73 % of all etiologies, alcoholism was the
predominant cause of cirrhosis.

According to the Child-criteria the patients varied sub-
stantially: three times Child A, seven times Child B,
five times Child C. Only subjects with decompensated
cirrhosis were selected as possible adverse effects of
the ß-blockade were under investigation in these patients
at the same time.

As to this point, data are not sufficient yet for a
meaningful statement.

With one exception a single dose of glycerolnitrate sublingually applicated resulted in a decrease of the hepatic venous pressure. The magnitude of this effect amounted to 20 % and was in the same range of that achieved
with ß-blockers (1, 2, 3, 4). As the data represent the
acute effect, future clinical trials are necessary to
establish, whether intravenous infusions in acute oesophageal variceal bleeding or if administration of retard
preparations for prophylaxis are of therapeutical value.
These investigations are in progress. As to therapy of
acute bleeding, clinical experience is limited to a trial
with a combination of vasopressin and nitroglycerin (5).
Nitroglycerin enhanced slightly the effect of vasopressin
to lower portal venous pressure and suppressed some side
effects of vasopressin. Direct measurements of the
pressure with oesophageal varices demonstrated a decrease
of pressure by 50 % (6), which appears rather high as
compared to our results. Our data are not in accordance
with observations of GIBSON and coworkers (7), who found
that only orally administered but not sublingually
applicated nitroglycerin decreased portal pressure. At
this point data are not sufficient to allow an explanation of the mechanism of action. Possibly the drop of
cardiac output causes a decreased portal blood flow, as
actually measured by FEELY (8).

As repeatedly shown (1, 2), ß-blockers lead to lowered portal pressure. The data in this investigation are compatible with this observation. The small number of subjects including two non-responsive patients is probably the reason for the lack of statistical significance. It seems important to note that the effect of nitroglycerin was additive to that of ß-blockers, which is documented by the lowered heart rate. Both substances together led to a decrease of the pressure by about 40 %. These data suggest that both substances have different mechanisms of action although there is no information as to which.

In conclusion nitroglycerin has a reproducible ability to lower the portal blood pressure acutely by about 20 %. The action is additive to that of ß-blockers resulting in a decrease of portal pressure by about 40 %. Further investigations are necessary to demonstrate the benefit no nitroglycerin in the therapy and prophylaxis of oesophageal variceal bleeding.

References

1. Bützow, G.H., Remmecke, J., Bräuer, A. (1982). Metoprolol in portal hypertension. A controlled study. Klin. Wochenschr. 60, 1311-1314

2. Lebrec, D., Nouel, O., Corbic, M., Benhamou,J.P.(1980). Propranolol - a medical treatment for portal hypertension? Lancet 2, 180-182

3. Burroughs, A.K., Jenkins, W.J., Sherlock, S., Dunk,A., Walt, R.P., Osnafor, T.O.K., Mackie, S., Dick, R. (1983). Controlled trial of propranolol for prevention of recurrent variceal hemorrhage in patients with cirrhosis. N.Engl. J. Med. 309, 1539-1542

4. Westaby, D., Bihari, D.J., Gimson, A.E.S., Crossley, I.R., Williams, R. (1984). Selective and non-selective beta blockade in the reduction of portal hypertension in patients with cirrhosis and portal hypertension. Gut 25, 121-124

5. Groszmann, R.J., Kravetz, D., Bosch, J., Glickman, M., Bonix, J., Bredfeldt, J., Conn, H.O., Rodes, J., Storer, E.H. (1982). Nitroglycerin improves the hemodynamic response to vasopressin in portal hypertension. Hepatology 2, 757-762

6. Staritz, M., Poralla, T., Ewe, K., Meyer zum Büschenfelde, K.-H. (1984). Der Einfluß von Nitroglycerin auf den Oesophagusvarizendruck bei Patienten mit Leberzirrhose. Z. Gastroenterol. 22, 423

7. Gibson, P.R., Mclean, A.J., Jakobowitz, A.W., Dudley, F.J. (1982). Medical management of portal hypertension: hypothesis and preliminary investigations. Gut 23, A 432-463

8. Feely, J. (1984). Nifedipine increases and glycerol trinitrate decreases apparent liver blood flow in normal subjects. Brit.J.Clin.Pharmacol. 17, 83-85

Reprints to:

Priv.-Doz.Dr.med. G.Bützow
Med. Kernklinik und Poliklinik
Universitäts-Krankenhaus Eppendorf
Martinistr. 52

D - 2000 Hamburg 20

14

The Effect of Glyceryl Trinitrate on the Intravascular Oesophageal Variceal Pressure in Patients with Cirrhosis and Portal Hypertension

M. STARITZ, T. PORALLA, T. HÜTTEROTH and
K.H. MEYER ZUM BÜSCHENFELDE

1st Medical Department, Johannes Gutenberg University Mainz

Zusammenfassung

Glyceroltrinitrat (GTN) führt zur Erschlaffung der glatten Muskulatur von Blutgefäßen. Es wurde daher für möglich gehalten, daß es den Pfortaderhochdruck bei Patienten mit Leberzirrhose vermindern könnte.

Mit der kürzlich beschriebenen endoskopischen Feinnadelpunktion von Ösophagusvarizen konnte der Einfluß von GTN auf den intravasalen Ösophagusvarizendruck (IOVD) gemessen werden. Drei Minuten nach sublingualer Gabe von 2.2 mg GTN fiel der IOVD bei 10 Patienten mit Varizen Grad III von 22.8 ± 2.0 mmHg auf 12.0 ± 0.4 mmHg ($p < 0.005$) und bei sechs Patienten mit Varizen Grad II von 16.3 ± 0.4 mmHg auf 10.0 ± 0.4 mmHg ($p < 0.005$).

Unsere bisherigen Ergebnisse lassen vermuten, daß GTN zur Blutstillung bei der Ösophagusvarizenblutung geeignet sein könnte.

Weitere Studien sollten darüber Aufschluß geben, ob Langzeitnitrate auch zur Prophylaxe der Varizenblutung geeignet sind.

Key words: Intravascular oesophageal variceal pressure, portal hypertension, endoscopic oesophageal variceal manometry, glyceryl trinitrate

Introduction

The prophylaxis of oesophageal haemorrhage by using beta
adrenal receptor blocking drugs has attracted widespread
attention. After first enthusiastic reports (1,2), however, further clinical trials were unable to detect any
benefit (3).

One carefully designed study including propranolol,
atenolol, and prazosine demonstrated that following application of these agents the gradient between free and
wedged hepatic pressure was lowered only to a small amount
of approximately 3 mmHg (4).

Since GTN is known to relax smooth muscles of vessels, it
was considered to reduce portal hypertension, too. Some
recent studies tried to evaluate this hypothesis, but
their results were conflicting, presumably mainly due to
the lack of a method providing exact estimation of the
variceal pressure. GROSSMANN (5) and FREEMAN (6) found
beneficial effects in this respect, DAWSON (7) and HALLE-
MANS (8) did not.

Therefore we re-evaluated the effect of GTN on oesophageal variceal pressure using a recently developed procedure which allows direct measurement of the IOVP (9).

Our study clearly demonstrates that GTN significantly
lowers the IOVP. The presumed clinical relevance of this
effect is discussed.

Methods

Patients

16 patients (9 male, 7 female, mean age 54 years, range
40 - 63 years) with histologically proven cirrhosis
(Child A) were included in the study. All of them had
previously bled from oesophageal varices at least 3 days
prior to the investigation. At the time of the study
systolic arterial blood pressure exceeded 100 mmHg in all
patients. Four patients were on treatment with Spirono-
lactone (50 mg/day). The application of adreno receptor

blocking agents or other drugs with presumed effect on portal hypertension was anamnestically excluded. Informed written consent was obtained from all patients.

At the time of the study inspection with a flexible endo-scope (Olympus GIF-Q) revealed no acute haemorrhage in the duodenum, stomach, and oesophagus. The oesophageal variceal columns were graded subjectively by an experien-ced endoscopist according to the classification reported by PAQUET (10). Spontaneously visible variceal columns in the lower and medium third of the oesophagus were classi-fied as grade II (n=6) and large variceal columns nearly occluding the oesophageal lumen as grade III (n=10).

Manometric examination

For the manometric examination a commercially available endoscopic sclerosing probe (Olympus) was passed through the channel of the endoscope. The inner lumen of the probe was perfused via a Statham element (BECKMAN R 427 G) using a hydraulic perfusion pump according to ARNDORFER (11) with a constant perfusion volume of 0.2 ml saline/ min. The pressure obtained at the tip of the needle could be recorded by a writer on a paper running with a speed of 1 mm/sec.
Each manometric examination started with recording of the oesophageal pressure by positioning the tip of the needle free in the oesophageal lumen. Then the oesophageal varices were punctured by the fine needle (diameter 0.71 mm) 10 cm proximally to the cardia and the intravascular pressure was obtained. After this, 1.2 mg GTN (Nitro-Lingualspray, Pohl-Boskamp, Hohenlockstedt, W-Germany) was sprayed into the tongues of the patients. Three minutes later the manometric examination was repeated as described above. The IOVP was estimated taking the pressure in the oesophageal lumen as zero-reference. All values are reported as mean $\pm$ SEM. For statistical analy-sis of the pressure values obtained before and after GTN application the Wilcoxon test was used.

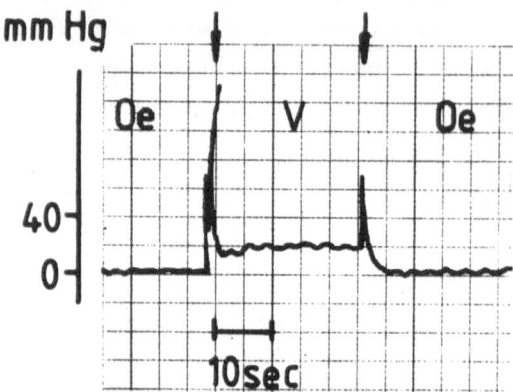

Fig. 1: Original tracing of the pressure in the lumen of
        the oesophagus (Oe) and the variceal lumen (V).
        The IOVP is calculated taking the pressure in the
        oesophageal lumen as zero-reference.

Results

In the lumen of the oesophagus and the variceal columns
small respiratory pressure alterations were recorded not
exceeding the amount of 4 mmHg (fig. 1).
IOVP in varices grade II amounted to 16.3 ± 0.4 mmHg and
in varices grade III to 22.8 ± 2.0 mmHg respectively
(fig. 2). IOVP obtained 3 minutes after the application
of GTN was reduced in all patients. It amounted to
10.0 ± 0.4 mmHg in grade II and 12.0 ± 0.4 mmHg in grade
III varices respectively (fig. 2, p 0.005, when compared
to pre-treatment values in both groups).

We did not observe any complications due to the diagnostic
variceal puncture. After retraction of the fine needle out
of the variceal lumen the endoscope was immediately passed
through the cardia for approximately 3 minutes. Under
these conditions only minute amounts of blood were oozing
from the site of the puncture.

Discussion

Previous methodical evaluations of this method for
assessment of IOVP clearly demonstrated the reliability
and safety of the method and the reproducibility of the
results (9). Meanwhile we have performed this procedure

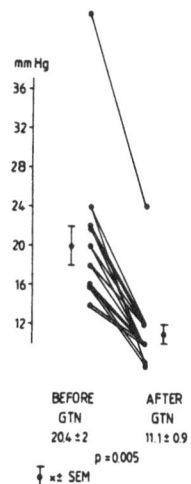

Fig. 2: Effect of glyceryltrinitrate (GTN) on the IOVP. Each line connects the IOVP obtained before and after application of GTN in one individual patient.

more than 100 times and observed not any complications. Particularly no variceal haemorrhage was caused by the diagnostic puncture. The advantage of the method lies in the fact that it provides exact direct measurement of the intravascular oesophageal pressure very close to the area where variceal bleeding usually occurs. Thereby the required technical equipment is easily available and the procedure may be performed without difficulties by endoscopists familiar with endoscopic sclerosing technique (12).

In contrast it is not yet proven that other procedures such as estimation of the free and wedged hepatic pressure (13) sufficiently correlate with the pressure inside oesophageal varices, the risk of further haemorrhage and the size of the varices. Furthermore, several investigators failed to detect a correlation between portal pressure and the risk of variceal haemorrhage (14, 15). The results reported by BURROUGHS and coworkers (3) who found that despite diminished portal pressure due to the

application of propranolol the incidence of further
variceal bleeding in treated patients was as great as in
the placebo group, may cast further doubt whether portal
pressure - or the difference between wedged and free
hepatic pressure - is a reliable parameter for studying
the effect of drugs with presumed therapeutic or prophylactic benefit in variceal haemorrhage.

Our study showed GTN to reduce the pressure in
oesophageal varices to approximately 50 % of its basal
pressure. Due to the short half life of 5 minutes (16)
this reported effect of GTN should be transient and
therapeutic applicability certainly depends on maintenance of appropriate drug levels over a longer period
of time. In our intensive care unit this aim was achieved
by using continuously intravenous infusion therapy of
GTN (5 mg/hour). In this way severe bleeding from varices
just below the cardia in two patients with oesophageal
varices grade III and pronounced fundus varices in whom
the Linton-Nachlas tube was only partially effective, was
stopped. In these patients IOVP dropped from 24 and 22 mm
Hg to 4 and 8 mmHg respectively under intravenous GTN-
administration.

In our opinion these experimental data and the preliminary
clinical results warrant further studies including a
greater number of patients to define the role of GTN in
the treatment of variceal haemorrhage in comparison with
other more established approaches such as application of
balloon tamponade, vasopressin treatment and sclerotherapy.
Furthermore, the impressive short term effectivity of
GTN in lowering IOVP as demonstrated in our study should
induce evaluations of the effect of longer acting
nitrates on IOVP.

References

1. Lebrec, D., Nouel, O., Bernuae, J., Bouygues, M.,
   Rueff, B., Benhamou, J.P. (1981). Propranolol in pre-

vention of recurrent gastrointerstinal bleeding in
cirrhotic patients. Lancet 1, 1920-21

2. Lebrec, D., Poynard, T., Hillon, P., Benhamou, J.P.
   (1981). Propranolol for prevention of recurrent
   gastrointestinal bleeding in patients with cirrhosis.
   N. Engl. J.Med. 305, 1371-74

3. Burroughs, A.K., Jenkins, W.J., Sherlock, S. (1983).
   Controlled trial of propranolol for the prevention of
   recurrent variceal hemorrhage in patients with
   cirrhosis. N. Engl.J.Med. 309, 1539-42

4. Mills, P.R., Rae, A.P., Farah, D.A., Russell, R.I.,
   Lorimer, A.R., Carter, D.C. (1984). Comparison of three
   adrenoreceptor blocking agents in patients with cirrhosis and portal hypertension. Gut 25, 73-78

5. Groszmann, R.J., Kravetz, D., Bosch, J. (1982).
   Nitroglycerin improves the hemodynamic response to
   vasopressin in portal hypertension. Hepatology 2,
   757-62

6. Freeman, J.G., Barton, J.R., Record, D.D. (1983).
   Effects of vasodilators on portal pressure in patients
   with portal hypertension. Gut 24, A 971

7. Dawson, J., West, R., Gertsch, P., Mosimann, F.,
   Elias, E. (1983). Endoscopic variceal pressure measurements: Response to isosorbite dinitrate. Gut 24, A 971

8. Hallemans, R., Naeije, R., Mols, P., Melot, C.,
   Reding, P. (1983). Treatment of portal hypertension
   with isosorbite dinitrate alone and in combination
   with vasopressin. Crit. Care Med. 11, 536-40

9. Staritz, M., Poralla, T., Meyer zum Büschenfelde, K.H.
   Direct oesophageal variceal pressure assessed by intra-
   variceal endoscopic manometry. (Gut, in press)

10. Paquet, K.J. (1982). Prophylactic endoscopic sclero-
    sing treatment of the oesophageal wall in varices -
    A prospective controlled randomized trial.
    Endoscopy 14, 4 - 5

11. Arndorfer, R.C., Steff, J.J., Dodds, W.J., Linehan,
    J.H., Hogan, W.J. (1977). Improved infusion system for

intraluminal oesophageal manometry. Gastroenterology
<u>24</u>, 7 - 23

12.Rose, J.D.R., Crane, M.D., Smith, P.M. (1983). Factors
affecting successful endoscopic sclerotherapy for
oesophageal varices. Gut <u>24</u>, 946-49

13.Boyer, T.D., Triger, D.R., Horisawa, M., Redeker, A.G.,
Reynolds, T.B. (1977). Direct transhepatic measurement
of portal vein pressure using a thin needle.
Gastroenterology <u>72</u>, 584-89

14.Mc Leod, M.K., Eckhauser, F.E., Turcotte, J.G. (1981).
Significance of corrected sinusoidal pressure (CSP)
in patients with cirrhosis and portal hypertension.
Ann. Surg. <u>194</u>, 562-67

15. Lebrec, D., de Fleury, P., Rueff, B., Nahum, H.,
Benhamou, J.P. (1980). Portal hypertension, size of
oesophageal varices, and risk of gastrointestinal
bleeding in alcoholic cirrhosis.
Gastroenterology <u>79</u>, 1332-39

16. Armstrong, P.W., Armstrong, J.A., Marks, G.S. (1979).
Blood levels after sublingual nitroglycerin.
Circulation <u>59</u>, 585-88

Reprints to:

Dr. Martin Staritz
I. Med.Klinik und Poliklinik der Universität Mainz
Langenbeckstraße 1

D - 6500 Mainz, FRG

15

Is the Beta Blocking Agent Metipranolol able to Reduce the Frequency of Recurrences After Endoscopic Sclerosis because of Bleeding Esophageal Varices?

K.-J. PAQUET, H. FEUSSNER and P. KOUSSOURIS

Department of Surgery, Heinz Kalk Klinik Bad Kissingen, W. Germany

Zusammenfassung

LEBREC und Mitarbeiter konnten in einer prospektiven kontrollierten randomisierten Studie durch Anwendung des Betablockers Propranolol, der die Herzfrequenz um mindestens 25 % senkte, die Häufigkeit von Blutungsrezidiven nach Ösophagusvarizenblutung bei CHILD A-Patienten signifikant senken. Diese kontrollierte Untersuchung konnte bei einem nicht ausgewählten Krankengut bisher nicht bestätigt werden. Aus diesem Grund sollte in einer prospektiven kontrollierten randomisierten Studie überprüft werden, ob Metipranolol, das durch die Leber besser verstoffwechselt wird als Propranolol, in einer Dosierung, die die Herzfrequenz um mindestens 25 % senkt, in der Lage ist, die Blutungsrezidivquote von 10 - 15 % nach erfolgter Wandsklerosierung der Speiseröhre wegen rezidivierender Ösophagusvarizenblutung und unter ständiger endoskopischer Kontrolle und Resklerosierung weiter zu senken. 102 Patienten wurden nach einer Randomliste in die Studie aufgenommen und in zwei Gruppen unterteilt. Sie unterschieden sich nicht in wesentlichen Kriterien wie Alter, Geschlechtsverteilung, Zahl der erhaltenen Bluttransfusionen, der vorausgegangenen Varizenblutungen, den Ursachen der Zirrhose, den endoskopisch gesicherten

Blutungsquellen, den biochemischen Leberfunktionsproben
und dem CHILD-Stadium. 14 Patienten der Placebo-Gruppe
(27 %) und 16 (32 %) der Substanzgruppe mußten aus verschiedenen Gründen aus der Studie ausgeschlossen werden.
Die Rezidivrate der endoskopisch nachgewiesenen Blutungen
aus Ösophagusvarizen und Magenerosionen betrug in der
Placebo-Gruppe 7,6 und in der Substanzgruppe 14 %; dieser
Unterschied ist statistisch signifikant zugunsten der
Placebo-Gruppe. Demnach ist es nicht berechtigt, Patienten zur Verhütung von Blutungsrezidiven nach Ösophagusvarizenblutung einen Beta-Blocker zu verabreichen.

Propranolol given orally in dosis that would reduce the
heart rate by 25 % in contrast to placebo administration
decreased corrected sinosoidal pressure and was able in a
controlled study conducted by LEBREC to reduce recurrent
gastrointestinal hemorrhage in patients with liver cirrhosis and esophageal varices significantly (1 - 3). A
controlled trial of propranolol conducted by BURROUGHS
et al. in London showed contradictory results (6).

Because from these and other studies it could not be
concluded that propranolol was a safe drug to prevent
recurrent hemorrhage in patients with liver cirrhosis and
portal hypertension we decided to make a different
schedule for a controlled trial. From June 1st, 1982, to
June 1st, 1983, metipranolol which is better metabolized
by the liver than propranolol was studied in a controlled
trial in patients with liver cirrhosis and portal hypertension which had been pretreated at least by one phase
of sclerotherapy during or after an active bleeding from
esophagogastric varices. 102 patients were randomly
assigned to two groups under the following criteria
(Tab. 1).

Material and Methods
The main question of this controlled trial was, if metipranolol is able to reduce the recurrence rate of variceal

hemorrhage 10 to 15 % after endoscopic sclerosis and permanent endoscopic control and if necessary resclerosis (5). The two groups were similar in demographic characteristics, etiology and severity of cirrhosis, and clinical course and laboratory tests (Tab. 2).

Table 1: Criteria for inclusion into and plan of the controlled trial. 01.06.1982 - 01.06.1983 Heinz Kalk-Clinic, D-8730 Bad Kissingen, W.-Germany

1. Endoscopically proved hemorrhage from esophago-gastric varices

2. Classification of varices III - IV (according to PAQUET)

3. At least 3 units of blood should have been transfused.

4. At least one phase (2 - 5 sessions) of endoscopic injection sclerotherapy should be finished (10 - 15 % recurrent rate !).

5. The schedule of resclerosis should not be interrupted.

6. Stabilisation of clinical and hemodynamic parameters, usually ten days after hospital admission.

7. Twice a day 5 - 20 mg Metipranolol up to the reduction of heart rate to 25 %.

8. A placebo was given to the control group.

9. Patients and doctors didn't know which patients received placebo or drug.

Table 2: Clinical parameters of patients.

	Placebo	Substance
Number of patients	52	50
Age (median value and fluctuation)	47,4 (28-81)	48,3 (26 - 79)
Sex (male(female)	35/17	32/18
Number of blood transfusion	3,5	3,3
Frequency of variceal hemorrhage	2,3	2,0
Type of cirrhosis alcoholic	30 (58 %)	28 (56 %)
non-alcoholic	22 (42 %)	22 (44 %)
Child classification at the beginning of the trial A	14 (27 %)	13 (26 %)
B	29 (56 %)	30 (60 %)
C	9 (17 %)	7 (14 %)

Results

14 patients from the placebo group (27 %) and 16 patients
(32 %) from the substance group had to be excluded. The
causes of exclusion are summarized in Tab. 3, which under-
lines the compliance rate of placebo was 87 % and of metipranolol of 80 %, which in our mind is not ideal but
sufficient.

Table 3:   Causes of exclusion from the trial.

	Placebo	Substance
Side effect of the drug	0	4
Stop to take the drug	7	6
elective shunt operation	3	2
Death — liver cirrhosis	2	2
Death — other causes	2	2
Compliance rate	14 (27 %)	16 (32 %)
	45 (87 %)	40 (80 %)

The recurrence rate of endoscopically proven variceal
hemorrhage (Tab. 4) and gastric erosions was 7,6 % in
the placebo and 14 % in the substance group.

Table 4: Recurrence rate of endoscopically proven
         variceal hemorrhage.

	Placebo	Substance
Varices	3	6
Erosions	1	1
	4 (7,6 %)	7 (14 %)
		p ◄ 0,01

This difference is statistically significant in favour
of the placebo group (p ◄ 0,01).

Discussion

Thus by the application of metipranolol twice per day with the dose that was able to reduce the heart rate to 25 % it was not possible to reduce the recurrence rate of gastrointestinal hemorrhage after an endoscopic injection sclerotherapy of esophageal varices. Even under the protection of sclerosis and in spite of the fact that the patients were regularly endoscopically controlled there was a recurrence rate of 14 % in patients treated by the drug. - Before a beta-blocking therapy is introduced as a regular therapy of patients with liver cirrhosis, portal hypertension and recurrent variceal hemorrhage more studies are necessary to determine which catagory of patients can profit from this therapy. In the interim, however, it should be stressed that betablockade should not be considered acceptable therapy and may indeed compromise patients with cirrhosis by precipitating encephalopathy or impairing cardiac output especially at the time of recurrent bleeding.

References

1. Lebrec, D., Louel, A., Corbic,M., Benhamou, J.P. (1980). Propranolol - a medical treatment of portal hypertension? Lancet II, 180 - 183

2. Lebrec, D., Poynard, T., Hillon, P., Benhamou, J.P. (1981). Propranolol for prevention of recurrent gastrointestinal bleeding in patients with cirrhosis. A controlled study. N.Engl.J.Med. 305, 1371-1374

3. Lebrec, D., Hillon, P., Munoz, C., Goldfarb, G., Novel, O., Benhamou, J.P. (1982). The effect of propranolol on portal hypertension in patients with cirrhosis: a hemodynamic study. Hepatology, 2, 523-527

4. Hillon,P., Lebrec,D., Munoz,C.,Jungers, M., Goldfarb, G., Benhamou, J.P. (1982). Comparison of the effects of a cardio-selective and a non-selective beta-blocker on portal hypertension in patients with cirrhosis. Hepatology, 2, 528 - 531

5. Paquet, K.-J., Feussner, H. (1983). Ist der Beta-
   Blocker Metipranolol zur Prophylaxe von Blutungsrezidiven nach Wandsklerosierung der Speiseröhre wegen
   blutenden Ösophagusvarizen geeignet? Z.Gastroent.21,427

6. Burroughs,A.K., Jenkins,W.J., Sherlock, S., Dunk,A.,
   Walt, R.P., Osuafor, T., Mackie, S., Dick,R. (1983).
   Controlled trial of propranolol for the prevention of
   recurrent variceal hemorrhage in patients with
   cirrhosis. N.Engl.J.Med., 309, 15 - 19

Reprints to:

Prof. Dr. med. K.-J. Paquet
Department of Surgery
Heinz-Kalk-Klinik Bad Kissingen
D - 8730 Bad Kissingen

16
Portal Drainage for Small-bowel Grafts: A Requirement for Successful Small-bowel Transplantation?

W.H. SCHRAUT, K.K.W. LEE and V.S. ABRAHAM

The University of Chicago, Department of Surgery

Zusammenfassung

Die venöse Drainage von Dünndarmtransplantaten kann entweder in die Pfortader oder in die vena cava erfolgen. Während Pfortaderdrainage die physiologische Route darstellt und potentielle immunologische Vorteile (immunsuppressiver Effekt der Leber) bietet, ist die systemische Drainage operationstechnisch einfacher, aber beinhaltet eine partielle porta-systemische Fistel. Ehe die Dünndarmtransplantation zur klinischen Anwendung kommt, sollte geklärt werden, ob dieser partielle porta-systemische Shunt signifikant immunologische Vorteile aufgibt und zudem metabolische Nebeneffekte verursacht und Leberfunktion beeinträchtigt, wie es nach einer zentralen portocavalen Anastomose geschieht.

Orthotope und heterotope Dünndarmtransplantation mit portaler (PV-D) oder systemischer venöser Drainage (SV-D) wurde in den Rattenspezies LBN-F1-LEW (semi-allogen), BN-LEW (voll-allogen) und LEW-LEW (isogen) durchgeführt. Portal-venöse Drainage verzögerte die Abstossung des Dünndarmtransplantates signifikant auf 22.8 Tage $\pm$ 6.2 (N=12) im Vergleich zu SV-D (11.8 Tage $\pm$ 2.2; N=24). Innerhalb der BN-LEW Spezieskombination konnte ein solcher Effekt nicht festgestellt werden (PV-D: 15.5 Tage $\pm$ 5.3,

113

N=11; SV-D: 16.2 Tage ± 5.6, N=11). Dies bedeutet, daß
der immunsuppressive Einfluss der Leber (Filtration und/
oder Modifizierung von Antigenen im Leberparenchyma)
geringfügig ist; ausreichend, um die Abstossung semi-
allogener, nicht jedoch voll-allogener Dünndarmtransplan-
tate zu verzögern.

Im Vergleich mit PV-D (N=7), verursachten isologe (LEW-
LEW) orthotope Transplantate mit SV-D (N=8) eine signifikante Hyperammonämie (PV-D: 83 µg/dl ± 10, SV-D: 140 µg/
dl ± 22); zentrale portocavale Anastomose (kein Transplan-
tat): 560 µg/dl ± 149), und eine geringfügige Leber-
atrophie (Leber/Körpergewicht Verhältnis: SV-D, 2.6 %;
PV-D, 2.8 %; zentrale portocavale Anastomose, 2.0 %).
Serumproteine, Leberhistologie und der allgemeine Ernäh-
rungszustand sowie Wachstum blieben unbeeinträchtigt
durch den Typ der venösen Drainage des Transplantates.

Der immunologische Vorteil, realisiert durch PV-D, ist
geringfügig und würde nicht eine unbedingte Bevorzugung
von PV-D über SV-D verlangen. SV-D geht jedoch mit
hepatologisch-metabolischen Veränderungen einher, die,
insbesondere beim Patienten mit vorgeschädigter Leber
(z.B., durch totale parenterale Ernährung), nicht unbe-
rücksichtigt bleiben können. Unter diesen Umständen er-
scheint die Erhaltung der Dünndarm-Leber Achse in der
Dünndarmtransplantation notwendig.

Introduction

One of the unresolved issues surrounding small-bowel
transplantation is the uncertainty as to whether the
venous effluent of the allograft should be drained into
the portal vein or whether it may be conveyed into the
inferior vena cava. The need to resolve this issue is
prompted by two concerns. First, an expanding body of
evidence from general (1,2) and transplantation (3-5)
immunology suggests that the liver is an immunologically
competent organ and may have a mitigating influence on

the rejection of allografts. Second, portal venous drainage, although it requires a technically more demanding
porto-portal anastomosis (PP-A), constitutes the
physiologic route of venous outflow, and it avoids the
potentially detrimental metabolic effects of systemic
drainage (PC-A, via the inferior vena cava) which,
although technically more easily achieved, constitutes a
partial porto-caval shunt.

Material and Methods

We employed a rat model of small-bowel transplantation,
whereby the entire small bowel was transplanted as an
accessory heterotopic graft for study of allograft rejection, or as an orthotopic isograft in place of the
recipient's own small bowel so that we could study the
metabolic effects induced by the type of venous drainage
used.

The following experimental groups were formed:

1. Heterotopic small-bowel transplantation with either
   porto-caval or porto-portal anastomosis in the LBN-F$_1$
   -LEW (PC-A, N=24; PP-A, N=12) and the BN-LEW (PC-A,
   N=11; PP-A, N=11) strain combinations.

2. Orthotopic small-bowel transplantation in the LEW-LEW
   strain combination (isografts) with either PC-A (N=8)
   or PP-A (N=7).

3. Central porto-caval shunt (PC shunt) in LEW rats (N=15).

4. Normal controls (N=6).

Postoperatively, the general health (activity, weight) of
the rats was observed and the appearance of the entero-
stomies was inspected on a daily basis. In the rats with
isografts, serum ammonia and protein levels were measured
2 weeks and 4-6 months after the operation.

For determination of allograft survival times, the death
of the recipient due to acute rejection constituted a
clear endpoint, whereas the endpoint for delayed chronic
rejection was less well-defined, consisting of entero-

stomal fibrosis and shrinkage of the allograft into a
hard, palpable mass in the recipient's abdomen. All rats
with isografts survived and were sacrificed 6 months
postoperatively, and the liver weight was determined.
Specimens from all small-bowel iso- and allografts and
from the recipient's own tissues (liver, bowel) were
prepared for light microscopic examination.
All data were expressed as mean and standard deviations.
Statistical significance was determined with the Student
T-test.

Results

Effect of type of venous drainage on allograft rejection

Survival of allografts in heterotopic position: In the
LBN-F_1-LEW combination, the grafts with PC-A were rejected
acutely leading to host death, after an average of 11.8 $\pm$
2.2 days (Table 1). Portal venous drainage prolonged allograft survival significantly to 22.8 $\pm$ 6.2 days. In 9 rats,
this chronic rejection process did not interfere with the
animals' well-being, whereas in 3 rats rejection ran a
subacute course, terminating with their death after 14
to 16 days.
When LEW rats were recipients of BN grafts, both acute
and chronic rejection occurred unrelated to the type of
venous drainage used. There was no statistically significant difference in the mean survival times between the
PC-A (16.2 $\pm$ 5.6 days) and PP-A groups (15.5 $\pm$ 5.3 days).

Histologic appearance of the allografts: Upon microscopic
inspection, the acutely rejected LBN-F_1 grafts displayed
extensive necrosis with mucosal sloughing and occasional
patches of remnant villi. Marked infiltration of the
bowel wall by leukocytes was evident. The lymphatic
tissues of the grafts disclosed lymphocytic depletion
with absence of germinal follicles. Chronic rejection was
characterized by encapsulation and coalescence of the
allograft into a hard mass. These grafts demonstrated

Table 1: Survival times and mode of rejection of hetero-
         topic accessory small-bowel allografts.

	No. of Rats	Mean Survival ± SD (days)	Model of Rejection Acute	Chronic
LBN-F$_1$-LEW				
PC-A	24	11.8 ± 2.2	24	0
PP-A	12	22.8 ± 6.2	3*	9
BN-LEW				
PC-A	11	16.2 ± 5.6	6	5
PP-A	11	15.5 ± 5.3	7	4

*   Subacute rejection

fibrosis and thickening of the bowel wall. The mucosa was
replaced by granulation tissue, with sporadic preservation
of structures resembling villi. The mesenteric lymph nodes
and Peyer's patches of these grafts showed severe lymphocytic depletion with fibrosis.

The microscopic appearance of the BN allograft rejected
by their LEW hosts was similar to that seen in the LBN-F$_1$
allografts undergoing the comparable mode of rejection
(acute or chronic).

Metabolic effects induced by the type of venous drainage
used

Weight and general health of the animals: Rats which
received isografts with either type of venous drainage
gained weight at a normal rate (+40 % above the preoperative weight within 6 months). In contrast, 6 of the 15
rats with a PC shunt died of emaciation 3-4 weeks after
the operative procedure, and the surviving 9 rats lost an
average of 20 % of their preoperative body weight within
6 months. Observations of behavior showed that all rats
with a PC shunt were restless and wasted a great deal of
rat chow while feeding; this was in marked contrast to
the behavior of the normal rats and of those that had
received transplants.

Autopsy findings: At sacrifice, the liver weight (as

percentage of the total body weight) of recipients of a
small-bowel isograft with PP-A was equal to that of
normal rats. In recipients of grafts with PC-A, the liver
had undergone a moderate degree of atrophy (not statistically significant), whereas rats with PC shunts had a
significant reduction in liver weight in comparison to
all other experimental groups (Figure 1). All vascular
anastomoses were found to be patent. There was no evidence of portal hypertension.

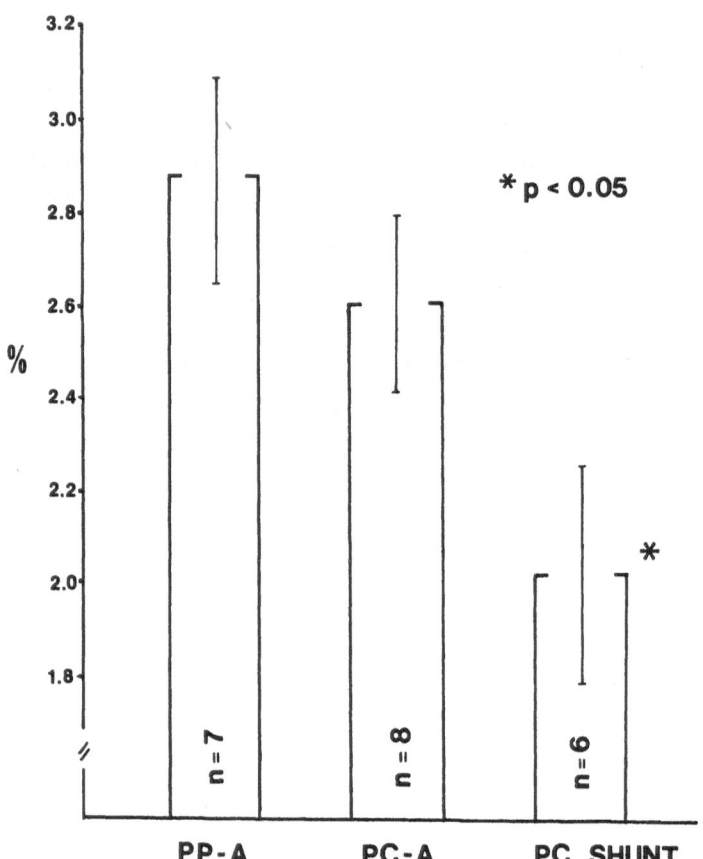

Figure 1: Liver weight as percentage of body weight in
rats 6 months after orthotopic small-bowel
transplantation (isografts) and after porto-
caval shunt. There is a statistically significant (P ◄0.05) reduction of the liver weight
between the shunted animals and those with
orthotopic isografts. The difference between
.the PP-A and PC-A groups is not statistically
significant.

Serum ammonia levels   (Figure 2): Serum ammonia levels
were the same for normal rats 84 µg/dl + 15) and for
those with isografts and PP-A (83 µg/dl + 10). Rats with
isografts and PC-A, however, developed significantly
elevated serum ammonia levels (140 µg/dl + 22) after the
operation. Rats with PC shunts became severely hyper-
ammonemic (560 µg/dl + 149) within 2 weeks after the
operation.

Serum protein electrophoresis: Albumin and globulin
levels remained unchanged in all groups throughout. the
6-month period of observation.

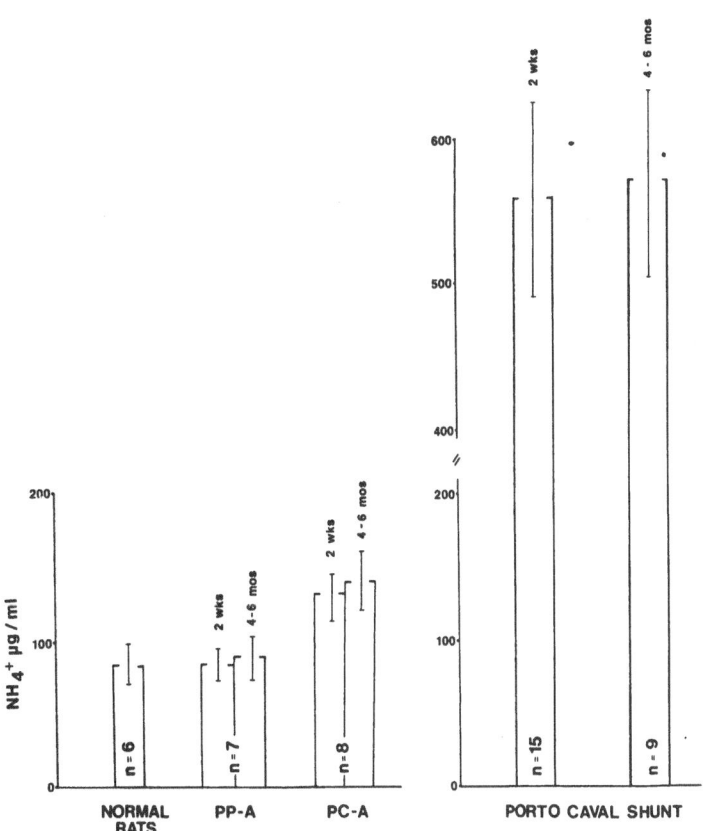

Figure 2: Serum ammonia levels after orthotopic small-
         bowel transplantation with either PP-A or PC-A.
         Ammonia levels are significantly higher
         (p◄0.05) in rats with a central porto-caval
         shunt and those with an intestinal isograft and
         PC-A when compared to normal rats and rats with
         orthotopic isografts and PP-A.

Histologic findings: Histologic examination of the isografts demonstrated an intact morphology. The livers of
the rats with isografts maintained a normal architecture
regardless of the type of venous drainage used. The liver
sections of the rats with PC shunts had a normal histologic appearance; there was no evidence of fibrosis.

Discussion

Our previous experience with small-bowel transplantation
(5) and the present experimental data demonstrate that
portal venous drainage alters and slows the rejection of
semi-allogeneic LBN-F$_1$ small bowel grafts by the Lewis
recipients. Both the experimental studies in rats by
BOECKX et al. (4) on cardiac allografts and by SAKAI (3)
on renal transplantation support our data. As to the
mechanisms that may underlie this immune-response-
modifying effect of the liver, several theories have been
proposed. SAKAI (3) and FREY et al. (6) suggest that the
transplantation antigens are degraded or filtered during
their passage through the liver, thereby reducing or
postponing stimulation of the host's immune system.
MANDEL et al. (2) suggested that an enzyme present in the
liver is responsible for inactivating transplantation
antigens or modifying circulating antigen reacting cells
thereby inhibiting an immune response.

Still, an exact understanding of the mechanism involved
remains elusive. Several studies on different organs and
different experimental models failed to demonstrate that
portal venous drainage alters or postpones allograft
(kidney, pancreas) rejection (7, 8); this may raise
doubts as to the existence of such an effect or, at least,
its importance and magnitude. The likely explanation for
the findings that are seemingly at variance with our
studies and with those noted above is that, in certain
species, the pancreas, kidney, and heart induce a strong
immune reaction within the host which prevents the
presumably weak immunosuppressive capacity of the liver

from being expressed in prolonged survival. This explanation is also supported by our finding that, in the BN-LEW
combination, which constitutes a match of great immuno-
geneic disparity, portal venous drainage failed to
influence intestinal allograft survival.

Thus, our investigations suggest that the immune-
response-modulating effect of the liver is a minor one;
it attenuates the rejection reaction of semi-allogeneic
(LBN-F$_1$) intestinal grafts only, whereas the rejection of
homozygous allogeneic (BN) small-bowel allografts remains
unaltered. Nevertheless, portal venous drainage may offer
benefits in terms of rejection control in clinical
practice. It is conceivable that the effects of portal
venous drainage would complement the immunosuppressive
drug regimens and thus reduce the doses needed for the
achievement of functional survival of small-bowel allografts.
Most investigators have utilized porto-caval anastomosis
rather than establishing normal physiologic portal
drainage for small-bowel allografts (9). If the use of
systemic drainage were to become standard practice, without regard to the potential, although minor, immunologic
benefits noted above, it should be recognized that
detrimental metabolic effects may arise. Our studies on
isografts indicate that selective shunting of the small-
bowel venous effluent is followed by metabolic alterations which are similar to those seen after total porto-
caval shunts (10, 11). However, these alterations are not
severe and appear to have no clinically observable
consequences. Nevertheless, with longer follow-up and
with the use of hepatotoxic immunosuppressive drugs,
these minor alterations (liver atrophy, hyperammonemia)
may evolve into real concerns in clinical small-bowel
transplantation. Moreover, many potential candidates for
small-bowel transplants, have received long-term total
parenteral nutrition, which is often accompanied by liver
impairment; this impairment might be ameliorated by an

increase in portal venous inflow provided by a small-bowel transplant with porto-portal venous anastomosis. Portal venous drainage may thus become the standard approach.

References

1. Cantor, H.M. and Dumont, H.E. (1967). Hepatic suppression of sensitization to antigen absorption into the portal system. Nature 215, 744

2. Mandel, M.A., Monaco, A.P., Russell, P.S. (1965). Destruction of splenic transplantation antigens by a factor present in liver. J. Immunol. 95, 673

3. Sakai, A. (1970). Role of the liver in kidney allograft rejection in the rat. Transplantation 9, 333

4. Boeckx, W., Sobis, H., Lacquet, A. et al. (1975). Prolongation of allogeneic heart graft survival in the rat after implantation on portal vein. Transplantation 19, 145

5. Schraut, W.H., Rosemurgy, A.S., Riddell, R.M. (1983). Prolongation of intestinal allograft survival without immunosuppressive drug therapy. J.Surg.Res. 34, 597

6. Frey, J.R., Geleick, H., DeWeck, A. (1964). Immunological tolerance induced in animals previously sensitized to single chemical compounds. Science 144, 153

7. May, A.G., Bauer, S., Leddy, J.P. et al. (1969). Survival of allografts after hepatic portal venous administration of specific transplantation antigen. Ann. Surg. 11, 824

8. Martin, X., Fraure, J.L., Amiel, J. et al. (1980). Systemic versus portal vein drainage of segmental pancreatic transplants in dogs. Transplant Proc.12,138

9. Kirkman, R.L., Lear, P.A., Madara, J.L. et al. (1984). Small intestine transplantation in the rat - Immunology and function. Surgery 96, 280

10. Herz, R., Sautter, V., Robert, F. et al. (1972). The Eck fistula rat: Definition of an experimental model. Europ.J.Clin.Invest. 2, 390

11. Lauterburg, B.H., Sautter, V., Preisig, R. et al. (1976). Hepatic functional deterioration after porta- caval shunt in the rat. Effects on sulfobromophthalein transport-maximum, indocyanine green clearance and galactose elimination capacity. Gastroenterology 71, 221

Reprints to:

Wolfgang H. Schraut, M.D.
The University of Chicago, Department of Surgery
5841 S. Maryland Avenue
Chicago, Illinois 60637, U.S.A.

17
The Effect of Portacaval Shunt on the $^{14}CO_2$-Exhalation from (Methyl-^{14}C)-Labelled Drugs

Ch. STEFFEN and O. ZELDER

Zusammenfassung

Die Abatmung von $^{14}CO_2$ aus (methyl-^{14}C)-markierten Arznei-mitteln wurde bei männlichen Wistar-Ratten 21 Tage nach portocavaler End-zu-Seit-Anastomose (PCA) gemessen. Einer Verminderung des Gehalts der Leber an Cytochrom P-450 um 70 % entsprach eine Abnahme der $^{14}CO_2$-Exhalation (CER) aus (Methyl-^{14}C)-Aminopyrin und -Antipyrin sowie eine Ver-längerung der Abatmungshalbwertzeit (CHL). Dagegen war die Abatmungsrate von $^{14}CO_2$ nach Sättigungsdosen von Methacetin (500 μmol/kg) nur um 30 % vermindert und die CHL nach 20 μmol/kg war von 30 auf 42 min verlängert. Hepatektomie nach PCA führte zu einer Senkung der CER auf 10 % des Kontrollwertes, so daß eine nennenswerte extra-hepatische Demethylierung von Methacetin ausgeschlossen ist.

Introduction

Alterations of liver perfusion by portacaval shunt will be followed by alterations of hepatic function, either directly by the diminished blood flow or subsequently by adaptive changes of hepatic tissue. As we were interested in changes of the drug metabolizing enzymes induced by portacaval end-to-side anastomosis (PCA), we measured the exhalation of $^{14}CO_2$ from a number of ^{14}C-labelled O- and N-methylated substrates in order to evaluate the mixed function oxidase of the liver. This method, the "breath test", is non-invasive, thus permitting the repetitive measurement of drug metabolism in the same animal which eliminates the large interindividual variations of cytochrome P-450 (1). Although the breath test with aminopyrine has been shown by LAUTERBURG and BIRCHER (2) to reflect changes of liver function caused by different methods including portacaval shunt, it is an indirect method an the correlation of ^{14}C-exhalation rate (CER) or ^{14}C-exhalation half-life (CHL) with the demethylation capacity remains to be established for each new substrate.

Material and Methods

The ^{14}C-labelled substrates antipyrine and aminopyrine were supplied by Amersham Buchler, labelled methacetin was synthesized as described by BRAUN et al. (3), cold methacetin by acetylation of anisidine (4), the other cold substrates were supplied by Merck, Darmstadt. The substrates were dissolved in saline or in polyethylene glycole (50 % in water) and injected intraperitoneally in a total volume of 1 ml. In the hepatectomy experiments both the control and the post-hepatectomy injection was given into the dorsal penis vein to avoid retarded absorption. 3-Methylcholanthrene (Eastman-Kodak) was dissolved in corn oil and injected i.p. (30 mg/kg body weight) 24 hrs before the experiment. Portacaval shunting was performed on male Wistar rats weighing 120 to 220 g as described previously (5), the measurement of $^{14}CO_2$ - exhalation and of cytochrome P-450 as described in (6). About 0.1 µCi of the labelled substrate was injected per animal. The CER is given as nmol of drug-derived CO_2 exhaled per minute, normalized to kg body weight.

Results and Discussion

Three weeks after PCA we could observe a significant decrease of liver wet weight from 10.5 $\pm$ 1.3 g (mean $\pm$ s.

d., n = 12) to 5.5 ± 1.1 g (n = 6) and a decrease of the
content of cytochrome P-450 from 700 ± 140 nmol/kg body
weight (n = 11) to 212 ± 118 (n = 6). The CER of aminopyrine was 30 % of the control value and the CHL was
prolonged by a factor of three. Similar changes are seen
with antipyrine, a hydrophilic substrate. Its CHL is
known to reflect the plasma half-life and is dose-inde-
pendent (7). After portacaval anastomosis, the CER is
diminished and the half-life is significantly prolonged
(Fig. 1).

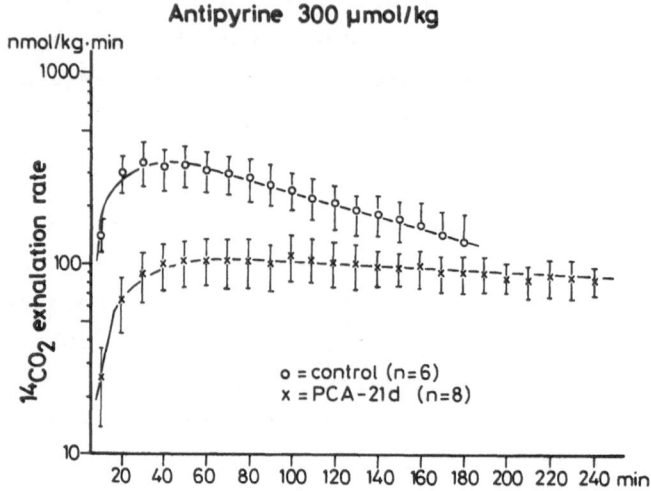

Fig. 1 : Drug-derived CO_2-exhalation rate (CER) in male
         Wistar rats after i.p. injection of (N-methyl-
         [14]C) antipyrine. Values are presented as mean ±
         s.d. 21 days after portacaval shunting the CER
         is decreased and the exhalation half- life is
         prolonged.

As one would expect that the metabolism of a drug with a
large distribution volume is dependent on liver blood
flow, we used the more lipophilic drug methacetin. When
this drug is used in a dose of 20 μmol/kg a maximum
CO_2-exhalation is reached after 30 min, and a half-life
of 27 min is seen (Fig. 2 and Table 1). After portacaval
anastomosis, the maximum value is diminished by 50 %, but
the CHL is only marginally prolonged. When saturation
doses are used the effect of PCA is even less expressed.

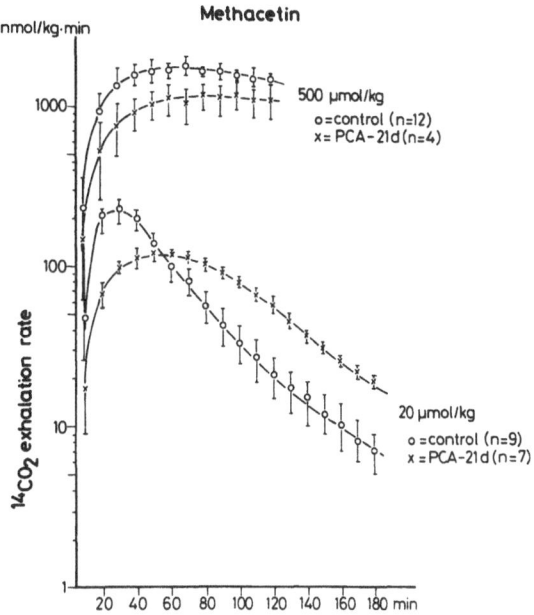

Fig. 2: Drug-derived CO_2-exhalation rate (CER) after
different doses of (methyl-^{14}C) methacetin in
male Wistar rats. The exhalation half-life
remains rather unchanged 21 days after portacaval shunting whereas the CER is decreased.

The different effects of PCA on the exhalation half-life
of the latter drug can be explained on the basis of the
observation that the serum half-life of methacetin is
much shorter than its exhalation half-life.
It could be shown that the CHL after methacetin in the
rat is independent of an induction by either 2-methyl-
cholanthrene or phenobarbital although both inducers show
distinct effects on the serum half-life which is shorten-
ed from the normal value of about 17 min to less than 10
min (8). The inductive effects of pretreatment, however,
are seen in the maximum exhalation rate after saturation
doses. With PCA, the diminution of the CER is rather small
in comparison to the large decrease of cytochrome P-450.
Two explanations for this effect were considered: A
relative increase of a methacetin-specific form of cytochrome P-450 or an extrahepatic metabolism of methacetin.

Table 1: Drug-derived CO_2-exhalation rate (CER) and -half life (CHL) after i.p.injection of (methyl-^{14}C) - labelled drugs in male Wistar rats before and 18 - 22 days after portacaval end-to-side anastomosis. Values are given as mean $\pm$ s.d., the number of animals is given in brackets. When saturation doses were used, a value for the CHL cannot be given.

	Controls		Portacaval anastomosis	
	CERmax	CHL	CERmax	CHL
	(nmol/kg min)	(min)	(nmol/kg min)	(min)
METHACETIN				
20 µmol/kg	224 $\pm$ 43 (9)	30 $\pm$ 1,7 (9)	111 $\pm$ 9,3 (6)	41,6 $\pm$ 8 (6)
500 µmol/kg	1650 $\pm$ 180 (12)	saturation	1100 $\pm$ 200 (4)	saturation
ANTIPYRINE				
300 µmol/kg	341 $\pm$ 88 (6)	134 $\pm$ 35 (6)	119 $\pm$ 18 (6)	335 $\pm$ 131 (6)
AMINOPYRINE				
100 µmol/kg	640 (2)	35 (2)	187 $\pm$ 22 (5)	118 $\pm$ 12 (5)

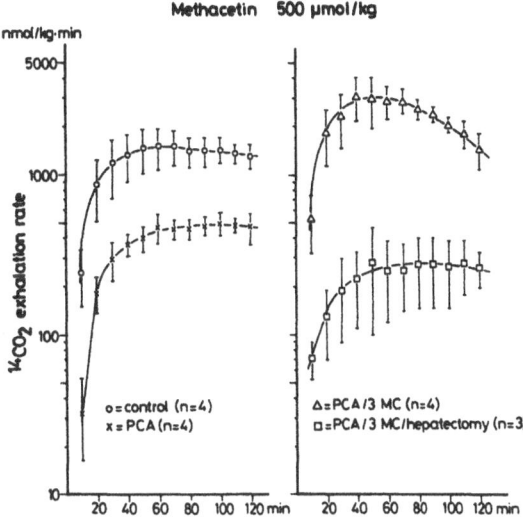

Fig. 3: Drug-derived CO_2 -exhalation rate after intravenous injection of (methyl-^{14}C) methacetin.
Control experiments were performed 1-2 days before
and 3-5 days portacaval anastomosis (left side).
The same rats were given 3-methylcholanthrene i.
p. and a breath test was performed 24 hours later.
After 4 days, induction was repeated and the rats
were hepatectomized (right side).

To exclude the latter possibility 4 rats (Fig. 3) were
tested with a saturation dose of methacetin before and
two days after PCA.

The CER decreased by approximately 50 %. One week later,
the same animals received 3-methylcholanthrene which is
known to induce the metabolism of methacetin. This pretreatment approximately doubled the CER and the exhalation curve shows that the dose of 500 µmol/kg is no
longer in the saturation range. A week later, the same
pretreatment was performed and the animals were acutely
hepatectomized in ether anaestesia. Less than 10 % of the
drug-derived CO_2 was exhaled by the hepatectomized rats.
This implicates that the extrahepatic metabolism of
methacetin is quantitatively negligible.
These results show that the CO_2 -exhalation rate is a useful method of monitor changes of liver drug metabolism

after different forms of treatment. It is, however, important to have a profound knowledge of the properties of the drugs used for this purpose.

References

(1) Chang, S.L., Nelson, S.D., Levy, R.H. (1984). Correlation between antipyrine clearance and cytochrome P-450 level after phenobarbital induction in rat. Drug. Met.Disp. 12, 139-141

(2) Lauterburg, B.H., Bircher, J. (1976). Expiratory measurement of maximal aminopyrine demethylation in vivo: effect of phenobarbital, partial hepatectomy, partacaval shunt and bile duct ligation in the rat. J.Pharmacol. Exp.Ther. 196, 501-509

(3) Braun, R., Dittmar, W., Hübner, G.E., Maurer, H.R. (1984). In-vivo-Einfluß von Valtrat/Isovaltrat auf Knochenmarkzellen der Maus und auf die metabolische Aktivität der Leber. Planta Med. 1, 1-4´

(4) Lumière, A., Lumière, L., Barbier, H. (1905). Acétylation en solution aqueuse. Bull. Soc. Chim., 3^esérie, 33, 783-787

(5) Zelder, O. (1984). Microsurgery in the portal area of the rat. In: Olszewski, W. (Ed), Handbook of microsurgery, CRC Press Inc., Boca Raton, USA, 331-348

(6) Daniel, W., Friebertshäuser, J., Steffen, C. (1984). The effect of imipramine and desipramine on mixed function oxidase in rats. Naunyn-Schmiedeberg's Arch.Pharmacol. 328, 83-86

(7) Rhodes, J.C., Houston, J.B. (1983). Antipyrine metabolite kinetics in phenobarbital and ß-naphthoflavone-induced rats. Drug.Met.Disp. 11, 2: 131-136

(8) Steffen, C., Wittig, M. (1984). Effect of phenobarbital and 3-methylcholanthrene on blood kinetics of methacetin and $^{14}CO_2$ exhalation in rats. Naunyn-Schmiedeberg's Arch.Pharmacol. 325, Suppl, R 11

Reprints to: Dr. Christian Steffen, Institut für Pharmakologie und Toxikologie, Philipps-Universität Marburg, D - 3550 Marburg/Lahn, Lahnberge

18
Portal Hypertension and Hemorrhage from Esophago-gastric Varices – A Contraindication for Pregnancy?

P. KOUSSOURIS and K.-J. PAQUET

Department of Surgery, Heinz Kalk-Klinik, Bad Kissingen

Zusammenfassung

Der Nachweis einer Leberzirrhose oder eines prähepatischen
Blocks mit portaler Hypertension und Ösophagusvarizenblutung wird als absolute Kontraindikation für eine
Schwangerschaft angesehen. Durch die folgende Kasuistik
soll demonstriert werden, daß dies heute nicht mehr für
den prähepatischen Block gilt. In der Chirurgischen
Universitätsklinik Bonn und M Department für Chirurgie
der Heinz Kalk-Klinik Bad Kissingen wurden von 01.01.72 –
01.11.84 12 Frauen in gebärfähigem Alter zwischen 17 und
31 Jahren wegen eines prähepatischen Blocks und Ösophagusvarizenblutung bzw. Zustand danach behandelt. Bei 7 lag
ein prähepatischer Block mit und bei 5 ohne komplette
Thrombose des Pfortadersystems vor; alle Frauen hatten
mit einer Ausnahme mehr als einmal aus Ösophagusvarizen
geblutet. Bei 5 Frauen ohne komplette Thrombose des Pfortadersystems wurde eine elektive Shuntoperation vorge-
nommen; vor einer Schwangerschaft kam es bei einer Frau
18 Monate danach zu einem Blutungsrezidiv, das auf einen
Shuntverschluß zurückzuführen war. Diese Frau wurde ebenso
wie 7 andere einer wiederholten Sklerosierungstherapie
zugeführt; nach mindestens 2 – 3 Sklerosierungsphasen
wurde ebenso wie nach erfolgreicher Shuntoperation zur

131

Schwangerschaft geraten und während der Schwangerschaft
fiberendoskopisch im 5. Monat und kurz vor der Geburt der
Befund von Speiseröhre und Mageneingang kontrolliert und
falls notwendig die Sklerosierung wiederholt. Während der
Schwangerschaft und Geburt traten keine Blutungsrezidive
auf; die 13 Frauen konnten von 20 Kindern in 5 verschiedenen Krankenhäusern entbunden werden. Die Geburten ver-
liefen ohne medikamentöse Therapie oder Operation
komplikationslos; kein Kind zeigte Schäden. Damit ist
nachgewiesen, daß ein prähepatischer Block heute nicht
mehr als Kontraindikation für eine Schwangerschaft angesehen werden kann, wenn durch eine erfolgreiche Shunt-
operation oder durch wiederholte endoskopische Sklerosierung und Kontrolle während der Schwangerschaft und der
Geburt das Blutungsrisiko auf fast 0 % gesenkt werden kann.

Introduction

The existence of an intrahepatic block based on a liver
cirrhosis or a prehepatic block is up to now respected as
an absolute contraindication for pregnancy. There are no
new arguments to change this opinion in case of compensated or decompensated liver cirrhosis even if after
successful shunt-operation, devascularisation, dissection
or an endoscopic sclerosis there is no danger of recurrence of variceal hemorrhage. Is this true for patients
with prehepatic block without liver damage, too? How
should be our recommendations to women with a prehepatic
block after a successful shunt-operation ? Which possibi-
lities of consultation and treatment exist for women with
total obliteration of the portal system before or after
shunt-operation, so that a decompression and elimination
of esophageal varices is impossible ?

Material and Methods

From January 1st, 1972 to January 1st, 1984 12 consecu-
tive women aged 17 to 31 years were admitted because of
hemorrhage from esophagogastric varices; the cause of

portal hypertension was a prehepatic block with or without complete thrombosis of the portal system (Tab. 1);
7 patients with a complete thrombosis of the portal
system had 5 episodes of variceal hemorrhage with the
range from 3 to 10 and were treated by emergency or
elective and repeated endoscopic sclerotherapy.

Table 1: Prehepatic block and pregnancy.
          Department of Surgery, University of Bonn and
          Heinz Kalk-Clinic Bad Kissingen, W.Germany

          n = 12 (01.01.1972 - 01.11.1984)

Number	Underlying disease	Number of bleedings	Method to stop hemorrhage
7	prehepatic block with	5 (3-10)	Endoscopic sclerosis 8 (7)
5	without complete thrombosis of the portal system	2 (1-4)	meso-caval 2 spleno-renal 1 coronario-caval shunt 2

In 5 women a selective lieno-, hepatico-, mesenterico-
and indirect portography which was performed in all women
during the bleeding free interval, visualized a super
mesenteric, splenic or left gastric vein suitable for a
shunt-operation. This group of patients had 2 episodes
of variceal hemorrhage with a rate from one to four. In
two patients a mesenterico-caval or coronario-caval and
in one woman a spleno-renal LINTON-shunt were performed
during the bleeding free interval. The mesenterico-caval
shunt was constructed without a prothesis. Four shunt
operations were performed before and one during the
fourth month of pregnancy.

Results

The function of the shunts was controlled fourteen days
and two years postoperatively by selective angiography.
One woman bled from esophageal varices 18 months after

meso-caval shunt; selective indirect mesenterico- and
cavography demonstrated a shunt obliteration. Bleeding
from esophageal varices ceased spontaneously; treatment
was continued by endoscopic sclerotherapy under regular
endoscopic control and if necessary resclerosis. The
recurrent hemorrhage from esophageal varices took place
before pregnancy. In the resting four women the function
of the two coronario-caval one mesenterico-caval and one
spleno-renal shunt could be visualized on angiography. -
There was no episode of variceal hemorrhage in these 5
women during pregnancy.

To get pregnant was advised in the resting 7 women with
total obliteration of the portal system after at least
two or three phases of sclerotherapy - usually 2 - 4
sessions in weekly interval - had been completed. Fiber-
optic control during pregnancy was performed during the
fifth month and 1 - 3 weeks before the exact day of
delivery (Tab. 2).

Table 2:   Number of phases of sclerotherapy.

before	during pregnancy
3 (2 - 5)	0,4 (0 - 1)

Only in 3 women a resclerosis during the fifth month of
pregnancy was necessary; in no woman a resclerosis had to
be performed before delivery. There was no episode of
variceal hemorrhage in this group of now 8 women during
pregnancy; one woman of the shunt group was transferred
to the sclerotherapy group because the obliteration of a
mesocaval shunt. Delivery in all women took place without
using special drugs or operation. In all 20 babies were
born in five different hospitals (Tab. 3):

Table 3:   Number of deliveries per woman.

Method of treatment	Number of deliveries	Number of babies	Number of women
Shunt	2 x 1 1 x 2 1 x 3	7	4
Sclerotherapy	4 x 1 3 x 2 1 x 3	13	8

Total number of babies   20

all deliveries progressed without complication. The four women with a functioning shunt gave birth to 7 and the resting 8 women treated by sclerotherapy to 13 babies. In none of the 20 babies any damage could be detected after birth.

Discussion

The exsistence of a prehepatic blocker with or without a complete thrombosis of the portal system is respected not at all as a contraindication for pregnancy today. In case there is no complete thrombosis of the portal system an elective shunt operation can be performed with a success rate of 80 %. After these operations the esophageal varices have disappeared and no danger of variceal hemorrhage remained. If the prehepatic block is charac-terized by complete thrombosis of the portal system or this thrombosis has developped secondarily after shunt obliteration the danger of hemorrhage before pregnancy can be reduced to at least 90 % by repeated endoscopic sclerotherapy. Using fiberendoscopic control and eventually resclerosis during pregnancy and before deli-very this protection against recurrence of hemorrhage can be enlarged to nearly 100 %.

Reprints to: Dr. med. P. Koussouris
             Department f. Chirurgie u. Gefäßchirurgie
             HEINZ KALK-Klinik
             D - 8730   Bad Kissingen

Isolated Hepatocytes

19

Complementation of Enzyme Deficient Mutant Rats by Auxiliary Transplantation of Intact Hepatocytes: Continuous Monitoring of Hepatocyte Integrety by Scintigraphy

D. HENNE-BRUNS, K. FRAMMINGER, D. PAUL[1], T. ROTHE[2], W. LIERSE[3] and B. KREMER

Department of Surgery, [1]Department of Pharmacology and Toxicology, [2]Department of Radiology, [3]Department of Neuroanatomy, Universität Hamburg, F.R.G.

Zusammenfassung

Voraussetzung für den funktionellen Nachweis auxiliär transplantierter Leberzellen ist entweder die Aufhebung eines erblichen, metabolischen Defektes am Versuchstier oder aber die höhere Toleranz gegenüber toxischen Substanzen. Ferner müssen die Zellen histologisch nachgewiesen werden.

In unserer Versuchsserie an Ratten konnte gezeigt werden, daß mit dem szintigraphischen Nachweis auxiliär in die Milz transplantierter Leberzellen, ein kombinierter Funktions- und Lokalisationsnachweis möglich ist. Die Szintigraphie eignet sich daher zur wiederholten Funktionsprüfung transplantierter Hepatozyten.

Schlüsselworte:
Auxiliäre Leberzelltransplantation, Leberzellszintigraphie

Transplantation of isolated hepatocytes is a widely used model for investigations of immunosuppressive drugs, vitality and induction of proliferation of transplanted cells.

In most experiments the function of transplanted hepatocytes can be shown by higher tolerance of the animal to hepatotoxic drugs (4, 7, 8) or by the complementation of

a congenital enzyme deficiency (1, 5) with the transplanted non-mutant cells.

An important problem is the determination of the vitality
and quantity of the transplanted hepatocytes (9). In most
experiments the vitality and quantity is proved by histological examination (4, 5, 6, 7,, 8). Therefore, animals
have to be killed and tests could not be repeated in the
same animal.

We used a scintigraphic technique for repeated determinations of the localisation and function of grafted hepatocytes in the same animal.

Material and Methods

Animals: Male Fischer 344 rats (180 - 200 g), Wistar rats
(200 - 325 g) and UDP-glucoronyltransferase deficient
Gunn rats (365 - 425 g) supplied by the Zentralinstitut
für Versuchstiere Hannover and Proefdieren Centrum
Heverlee were used.

Experimental Protocol: Group I (Syngenic transplantation):
Isolated hepatocytes of Fischer 344 rats in single cell
suspension were transplanted into the spleen of 6 inbred
Fischer 344 rats.

Group II (Allogenic transplantation): Hepatocytes of
Fischer 344 rats were transplanted into the spleen of
Wistar rats. Some recepients received Cyclosporin A for
immunosuppression. 2 other animals of this group were
transplanted without any immunosuppressive therapy.

Group III (Allogenic transplantation): Isolated hepatocytes of Wistar rats were transplanted into the spleen of
6 Gunn rats. 2 control animals received an equal volume of
a saline solution. In this group all animals were immunosuppressed with Cyclosporin A.

In all groups the isotope study was done four weeks after
transplantation. Subsequently the animals were killed and
tissues examined histologically.

Preparation of hepatocytes: Hepatectomy was performed
under ether anesthesia. Hepatocytes were prepared accor-

ding to the collagenase digestive method of WILLIAMS (10).
Usually about 75 % of the cells were viable as shown by
Trypan Blue exclusion tests one hour after isolation.
Hepatocytes (2 x 10^7 - 2 x10^8) suspended in 1 ml Hanks
solution were injected into the spleen immediately after
laparotomy.

Immunosuppression: Cyclosporin A (Fa. Sandoz 5 - 10 mg/kg
daily) was administered to the rats one day prior to the
operation. Cyclosporin A blood levels were determined
daily and ranged from 300 - 700 ng/ml.

Bilirubin determinations: Bilirubin levels in Gunn rat
serum were determined spectrophotometrically as descibed
by JENDRASSIK and GROF (2). Bilirubin levels were determined one week prior to the operation and thereafter for
4 weeks in weekly intervals.

Scintigraphy was performed by intravenous administration
of 99 Tc-HIDA (N-2,6-dimethylphenylcarbamoylmethyl-
iminodiacetic acid) in a dose of 10 μ Ci/100 g body
weight (3).

Histological studies: Light microscopy examinations on
H.E. and PAS stains were done of all spleens.

Results

After intravenous administration of 99 Tc-HIDA the isotope accumulates in the hepatocytes (3). After a short
circulation time (1 - 2 min) the radioactivity increased
rapidly in the peripheral parenchyma of the liver (Fig.1,
curve A). The uptake of the radioactive material into
the liver tissue is followed by a continuous fall of
radioactivity corresponding to biliary excretion.
Different time course of radioactivity was observed in
the spleen (Fig. 1, curve B). In control animals the
radioactivity is not taken up by the spleen. In contrast,
in animals which were transplanted with hepatocytes the
uptake of radioactivity occurs during the first 3 minutes
and remains constant for 10 - 15 minutes post infusion as
shown by the plateau-like curve (Fig. 1, curve B). This

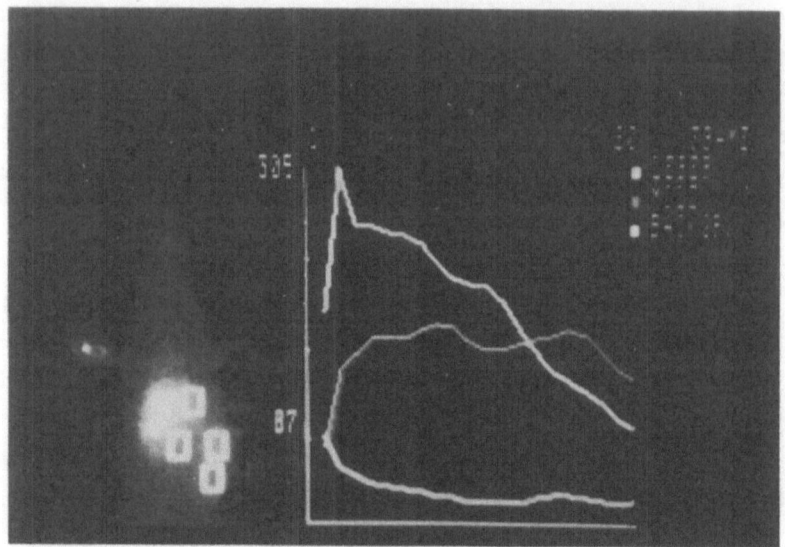

Fig. 1:   Time courses of radioactivity:
          A = liver parenchyma, B = transplanted hepato-
          cytes in the spleen, C = background

prolonged accumulation of the isotope presumably results
from the presence of radioactivity in transplanted
hepatocytes within the spleen and might be explained by
the lack of biliary excretion modus.

The lower curve (Fig. 1, curve C) represents the background radioactivity representing the isotope level in
the circulation.
These different time courses of radioactivity distribu-
tions allow us to differentiate between radioactivity in
the liver parenchyma and in transplanted hepatocytes.
Table 1 shows the results of our transplantation experiments in group I and II. The function of the transplanted
hepatocytes could be confirmed by scintigraphy and histological examination in all animals of group I (Fischer
344 rats). Function of transplanted hepatocytes could be
shown by scintigraphy and histological examination (Fig.
2) only in those animals of group II (Wistar rats) which
received immunosuppressive therapy (Table 1).

Table 1: Survey of results: Hepatocytes transplanted into
the spleen of Fischer 344 rats (group I) and
Wistar rats (group II).

Strain	Immunosuppressive Therapy	No	Scintiscan	Histology
Fischer (R)	-	1	+	+
Fischer (D)	-	2	+	+
	-	3	+	+
	-	4	+	+
	-	5	+	+
	-	6	+	+
Wistar (R)	+	7	+	+
Fischer (D)	+	8	+	+
	-	9	-	-
	-	10	-	-

D = Donor, R = Recipient

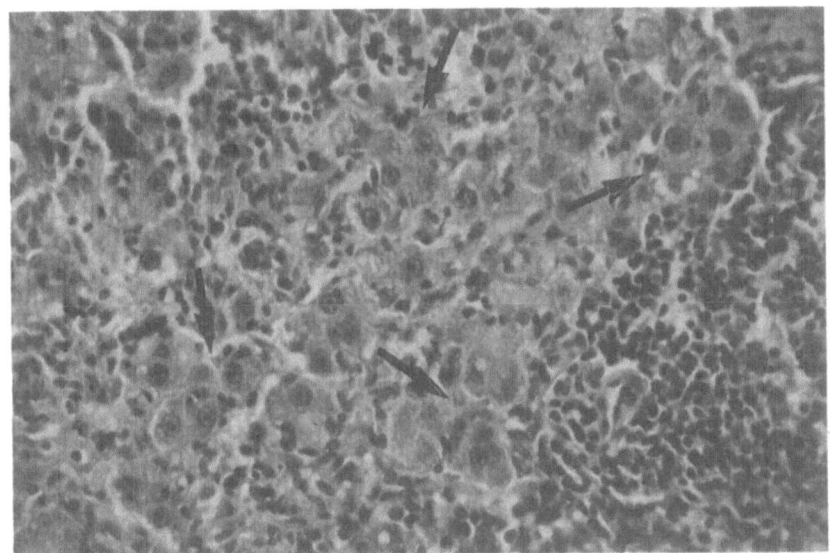

Fig. 2: Histology of transplanted hepatocytes in the
spleen of immunosuppressed Wistar rats four weeks
after transplantation (H.E. stain 1:300).

The function of the hepatocytes could be demonstrated by
the reduction of bilirubin levels and by scintigraphy in
animals of group III (Gunn rats, Table 2). Two rats of
these group died after 3 weeks (No 5 and 6, Table 2) and
isotope studies could not be performed. In two rats (No 7
and 8, Table 2) immunosuppressive therapy was terminated
four weeks after transplantation'. An isotope study two
weeks after termination of therapy did not show any
radioactivity in the spleen and the histological examination revealed the degeneration of the transplanted
hepatocytes (Fig. 3).

Tab. 2: Survey of results: Hepatocytes transplanted into
the spleen of enzyme deficient Gunn rats
(group III).

AUXILIARY LIVERTRANSPLANTATION			
4 weeks after transplantation			
Strain	No	Scintiscan	Histology	Reduction of Bilirubin
Gunn	1	–	–	3 %
(Control)	2	–	–	0,5 %
Wistar	3	+	+	30 %
to	4	+	+	24 %
	5	Ø	+	26 %
Gunn	6	Ø	+	31 %
	7	+	Ø	36 %
	8	+	Ø	27 %

Conclusion

A) Transplanted hepatocytes identified histologically in
the spleen in syngeneic recepient Fischer 344 rats can be
identified by scintigraphy due to the specific uptake of
Tc-HIDA in hepatocytes.
B) Allogenic control experiments (Fischer 344 hepatocytes
transplanted into the spleen of Wistar rats) showed that

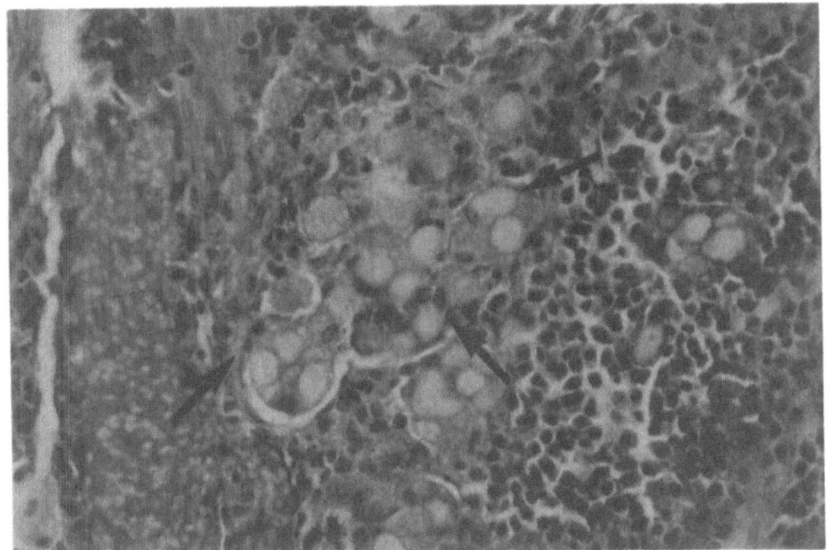

Fig. 3: Histology of transplanted hepatocytes in the
        spleen of Gunn rats 6 weeks after transplantation
        and 2 weeks after termination of the immuno-
        suppressive therapy. (H.E. stain 1:300) Vacuolar
        degeneration of the transplanted cells.

hepatocytes only survive in immunosuppressed recepients
as shown by histological and scintigraphical determinations.
C) Allogenic transplantation of Wistar hepatocytes into
immunosuppressed but not into untreated Gunn rat spleens
results in decreased bilirubin blood levels indicating
the intact function of the transplanted hepatocytes. The
presence of hepatocytes in the spleen was confirmed by
scintigraphy and by histological determinations.

References

1. Groth, C.G., Arborgh, B., Björken, C., Sundberg, B.,
   Lundgren, G. (1977). Correction of Hyperbilirubinemia
   in the Glucuronyltransferase-Deficient Rat by Intra-
   portal Hepatocyte Transplantation. Transplantation
   Proceedings 9, 313-316
2. Jendrassik, L., Grof,P. (1938). Vereinfachte photo-
   metrische Methode zur Bestimmung des Bilirubins.
   Biochemische Zeitschrift 297, 81-89

3. Loberg, M.D., Cooper, M., Harvey, E., Callery, P., Faith, W. (1976). Development of New Radiopharmaceuticals Based on N-Substitution of Iminodiacetic Acid. Europ.J. of Nuclear Med. 1, 137-139

4. Makowka, L., Falk, R.E., Rotstein, L.E., Falk, J.A., Nossal, N., Langer, B., Blendis, L.M., Phillips, M.J. (1980). Reversal of Experimental Acute Hepatic Failure in the Rat. J.of Surg. Research 29, 479 - 487

5. Matas, A.J., Sutherland, D.E.R., Stefes, M.W., Mauer, S.M., Lowe, A., Simmons, R.L., Najarian, J.S. (1976). Hepatocellular Transplantation for Metabolic Deficiencies: Decrease of Plasma Bilirubin in Gunn-rats. Science 192, 892 - 894

6. Minato, M., Houssin, D., Demma, I., Morin, J., Gigou, M., Szekely, A.M., Bismuth, H. (1984). Transplantation of Hepatocytes for Treatment of Surgically Induced Acute Hepatic Failure in the Rat. Europ. Surg. Research 16, 162 - 169

7. Mito, M., Ebata, H., Kusano, M., Onishi, T., Hiratsuka, M., Saito, T. (1979). Studies on Extopic Liver Utilizing Hepatocyte Transplantation into the Rat Spleen. Transplantation Proceedings 11, 585 - 591

8. Sommer, B.G., Sutherland, D.E.R., Matas, A.J., Simmons, R.L., Najarian, J.S. (1979). Hepatocellular Transplantation for Treatment of D-Galactosamin-Induced Acute Liver Failure in Rats. Transplantation Proceedings 9, 578 - 584

9. Woods, R.J., Fuller, B.J., Attenburrow, V.D. Nutt, L.H., Hobbs, K.E.F. (1982). Functional Assessment of Hepatocytes after Transplantation into the Rat Spleen. Transplantation 33, 123 - 126

10. Williams, G.M. (1977). Detection of Chemical Carcinogens by Unscheduled DNA synthesis in Rat Liver Primary Cell Cultures. Cancer Research 37, 1845-1851

Reprints to: Dr. D. Henne-Bruns
             Chirurgische Universitätsklinik Hamburg
             Martinistr. 52, 2ooo Hamburg 20, FRG.

20
Transfer of Hepatocytes and Cyclosporin A Therapy – Induction of Specific Tolerance?

G.H. MÜLLER, A. WUNDERLICH, U.T. HOPT and H. BOCKHORN

Chirurgische Universitätsklinik Tübingen

Zusammenfassung

Im starken Abstoßungsmodell der Ratte DA (Rt 1 a) zu
Lewis (Rt 1 l) werden Organtransplantate akut abgestoßen.
Cyclosporin A (CyA) verhindert diese Abstoßung und führt
zu einer Toleranz: Vaskularisierte Lebertransplantate (DA)
bewirken unter CyA-Therapie eine stabile Toleranz zu DA-
Nierentransplantaten. Im Gegensatz dazu wird keine Toleranz für spenderspezifische Zweittransplantate entwickelt,
wenn Leberzellsuspensionen unter Cyclosporintherapie in
die Milz transfundiert werden.

1. Introduction

The aim of transplantation immunology is still specific
immunosuppression. Such a therapy is as yet not available
for human beings; it can however be practised using
various methods in the rat model. We concentrated on two
phenomena, in order to study a combination of them in one
single form of therapy: we refer to liver transplantation
and CyA therapy. One result in particular arises from
either of these two processes; donor-specific tolerance.

Organ transplants are rejected in the rat model when
donor and recipient have different MHCs (major histocompatibility complexes). This does not apply in many

donor-recipient combinations in the case of orthotopic
liver grafts. Once the liver graft has been accepted, the
recipient develops a stable tolerance to donor-specific
secondary grafts (1, 2).

In the same strong rejection model, CyA prevents a rejection of vascularised organ transplants, admittedly only
for a short time. It also induces donor-specific tolerance,
which is maintained by suppressor cells (3). Pretreatment
of the recipient with antigenic material and CyA showed
that not only vascularised allotransplants lead to
transplant tolerance (4). The following experiments were
carried out in order to utilise the effect of suppressor
cell cloning, which leads to the induction of tolerance,
and combine it with the special immunological activity of
liver grafts.

2. Material and Methods

We used the strongrejection model DA (Rt - 1a) to Lewis
(Rt - 11). Male animals weighing between 175 - 250 g were
used. Cyclosporin was administered by gastric tube feeding
in doses of 10 mg/kg/body weight every day for 14 days.
Auxiliary liver transplants (5) and orthotopic kidney
transplants (6) were performed. Following portal vein
perfusion, liver cell suspensions were obtained using a
modified method (6); 50 minutes perfusion with 0.05 %
collagenase (clostridium histolyticum) and 0,1 %
hyaluronidase and Hank's Medium. A vitality test was
carried out. Hepatocyte suspensions with a cell count of
1×10^6 were injected into the spleen of the recipient
following a laparatomy. In each of the following experimental groups, 6 animals recieved transplants:

Group 1: Lewis without therapy, DA kidney

   2: Lewis + 14 days CyA; DA kidney on day 30

   3: Lewis without therapy, DA liver transplant

   4: Lewis + CyA + DA liver transplant

   5: Lewis + CyA + DA liver transplant; DA kidney on
      day 30

6: Lewis + DA hepatocytes + CyA for 14 days; DA
     kidney on day 30.

The day of rejection was taken as being the day on which
the animal died of uraemia following a contralateral
nephrectomy. The Wilcoxon test was used for statistical
analysis.

3. Results

Lewis recipients acutely rejected DA kidneys consistently
(Group 1). This was still the case after 14 days of CyA
pretreatment, followed by a DA kidney transplant after a
further two-week interval (Group 2). DA liver grafts were
just as acutely rejected by Lewis recipients. On day 14,
no living tissue could be observed. All the recipients
survived this rejection reaction. Using CyA therapy,
auxiliary liver transplants were not rejected. Histological examinations on days 14 and 30 showed, however, that
despite an intact structure, there were round cell infiltrations and the beginnings of atrophy of the transplant
(Group 4). When Lewis animals, with an auxiliary liver
graft and 14 days of CyA therapy, were given a secondary
transplant - a DA kidney - on day 30, they survived for at
least 70 days without rejection of the secondary transplant (Group 5). In contrast to this, all Lewis rats with
a secondary transplant following an initial hepatocyte
transfusion and untreated control animals died (Group 6).

Table 1:   Results - Lewis recipient survival

group (1)	11, 11, 12, 13, 13, 13
group (2)	12, 12, 12, 12, 13, 13
group (3)	6 x, rejection of liver grafts
group (4)	6 x 100 days, no rejection of liver grafts
group (5)	6 x 100 days, no rejection of kidney grafts
group (6)	12, 12, 13, 14, 14

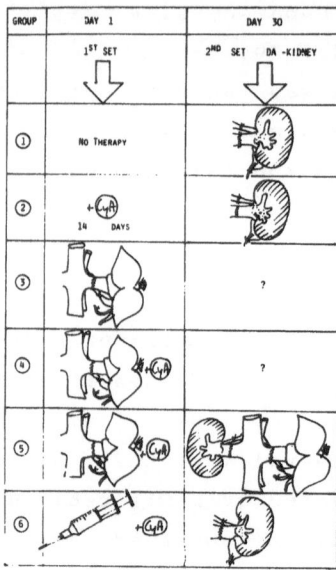

Fig. 1: Experimental Protocol - 1st set and 2nd set
         reaction in the DA to Lewis model after liver
         transplantation or transfer of liver cell
         suspension.

Discussion

The above studies reaffirm the peculiar immunological role
of the liver. They show donor-specific tolerance which is
typical both for liver transplantation and for treatment
with CyA. Although treatment with antigens led to a
change in the recipient's immunology in earlier experiments (4), no such effect was observed following trans-
fusions of liver cell suspension. The desired combined
effect of CyA and the specific effect of the liver was
not observed. The comparison of a vascularised liver
transplant with liver cell suspension showed several
significant differences. Although earlier tests showed
that hepatocytes could take over certain liver functions,
at least for a short while, a hepatocyte transfer is
immunologically scarcely comparable with vascularised
liver transplants. One reason for this is the modified
cell vitality, which changes the expression of the antigenic material. This is caused by perfusion-induced
ischaemia and enzyme fragmentation of the liver cell

suspension. Class I and II antigens characterize the liver. Only Class I antigens are found on the hepatocytes. Most of the class II antigens are to be found on Kupffer's cells. Both classes of antigens are important for the rejection reaction, whereby class II antigens display the highest antigenicity. We can only guess how important the intactness of the kupffer's cells is , which are transplanted in a live symplasm during liver grafting. In later experiments, an increased number of these cells has jet shown no change. This contrasts with our observation, that induction of tolerance is facilitated by an increase in the number of lymphocytes during Cyclosporin therapy. The quality of the antigens on the lymphocytes seems to be significant; B lymphocytes (class II of 1a antigens) seem better suited to induction of tolerance than T lymphocytes (8). There may be other methods, the specific elimination of donor-specific reacting T cells (clonal deletion) was discussed for the vascularised liver transplant. Opsonisation of alloreactive cells as a result of antigen excess is another hypothesis. The initial suppression of an immunological reaction is common to both CyA therapy and liver transplantation. It is possible that the lenght of duration of this mechanism is responsible for the creation of suppressor mechanisms, which maintain a specific tolerance.

References

1. Kamada, N., Davies, H.F.F.S., Roser, B.J. (1981). Reversal of transplantation immunity by liver grafting. Nature, 292, 840 - 842
2. Kamada, N., Davies, H.F.F.S., Wight, D., Culank, L., Roser, B. (1983). Liver transplantation in the rat: biochemical and histological evidence of complete tolerance induction in nonrejector strains. Transplantation, 35, 304 - 312

3. Hutchinson, I.V., Shadur, C.A., Duarte, A., Baldwin
   III, W.M., Strom, T.B., Tilney, N.L. (1981).
   Mechanisms of cardiac allograft prolongation by
   Cyclosporin A. Transpl.Proc. XIII, 412 - 416

4. Müller, G.H., Wunderlich, A., Hopt, U.T., Bockhorn,H.
   (1985). Spezifische Immunsuppression im Rattenmodell -
   erfolgreiche Empfängerkonditionierung mit Cyclosporin
   A vor Nierentransplantation.
   Langenbecks Arch. Suppl. 91 - 94

5. Müller, G.H. (1983). A simple technique for heterotopic auxiliary liver transplantation in the rat.
   Transplantation 36, 221 - 222

6. Müller, G., Fairbrother, B.J., Morris, P.J. (1982).
   Organ transplantation in the rat-kidney, heart,
   liver and pancreas transplants using the renal
   vessels. Langenbecks Arch. 358, 852

7. Berry, M.N., Friend, D.S. (1969). High yield
   preparation of isolated rat liver parenchymal cells.
   J. Cell. Biol. 43, 509 - 520

8. Müller, G.H., Wunderlich, A. (1985).
   in preparation

9. Davies, H.F.F.S., Kamada, N., Roser, B.J. (1983).
   Mechanisms of donor-specific unresponsiveness
   induced by liver grafting.
   Transpl. Proc. 15, 831 - 835

10. Roser, B.J., Kamada, N., Zimmermann, F., Davies,
    H.F.F.S. (1983). Immunosuppressive effects of
    experimental liver allografts. Liver Transplantation:
    The Cambridge King's College Hospital Experience
    (ed. R.Y. Calne). p. 35, Grune and Stratton

Reprints to:

Dr. G. H. Müller
Chirurgische Universitätsklinik Tübingen
Calwerstraße 7

D - 7400 Tübingen

21
Functional Assessment of Hepatocytes after Syngeneic Transplantation into Rat Spleen

H. LÖSGEN, T. YAMAMOTO*, T. KUSANO*, E. SCHMIDT, M. MITO* and G. BRUNNER

*Div. of Gastroenterology and Hepatology, Med. Hochschule, Hannover, F.R.G.; *Medical College, Asahikawa, Japan*

Introduction

Isolated hepatocytes transplanted into the spleen of rats proliferate. 6 - 24 months after transplantation a morpho- logical structure can be observed comparable to that of a normal liver. Only little is known on the functions of the ectopic liver in the spleen (1, 3). We therefore have investigated the activities of liver enzymes of different metabolic functions and intracellular localisation in the hepatized spleens.

Material and Methods

Enzymatically isolated hepatocites were transplanted into the spleen of male Fischer rats by the method of MITO et al. (1).
In two of six rats which showed hepatization of the spleen at exploratory laparatomy a portacaval shunt was done. 15 - 24 months after transplantation all animals were killed. The hepatized spleens were perfused with heparinized NaCl solution and on several sections the percentage of hepatic tissue in the spleen was evaluated.

The activities of GOT, GPT, GLDH, GDH and Cytochrome c reductase and the protein concentrations were determined

in the homogenate of livers, normal spleens and the
hepatized spleens by standard methods.

Abbreviations:

GOT: glutamic oxalacetic transaminase = aspartate amino-
     transferase EC 2.6.1.1. (cytosol. + mitochondr.
     enzyme)

GPT: glutamic pyruvic transaminase = alanine aminotransferase EC 2.6.1.2. (cytosol. enzyme)

GLDH: glutamic dehydrogenase EC 1.4.1.3. (mitochondr.
      enzyme)

GDH: glycerophosphate dehydrogenase EC 1.1.1.8. (cytosol.
      enzyme)

Cytochrome c reductase: NADPH-cytochrome c reductase
                        EC 1.6.2.4. (microsom. enzyme)

Results

The anatomical data of the animals and the amount of
liver tissue in the spleens are listed in Table 1. The
animals with portocaval shunt show reduced weights of
body, liver and spleen.

Table 1 :   Anatomical parameters in rats after syngeneic
            transplantation of hepatocytes into spleen.
            Animals No.1-4 without portacaval shunt.
            Animals 5 and 6 with portacaval shunt 10 months
            after transplantation of liver cells.

No.	time after Tx [months]	body weight [g]	liver weight [g]	spleen weight [g]	liver tissue in the spleen [%]
1	15	480	15,1	0,87	30-35
2	15	460	15,7	0,73	25-30
3	24	430	14,6	1,10	10-15
4	19	460	17,0	0,96	5
5	19	360	7,0	0,94	35-40
6	19	220	5,4	0,44	25-30

The specific activities of Cytochrome c reductase, GPT,
GDH, GOT and GLDH in normal livers, normal spleens and
hepatized spleens are summarized in Table 2 .
In the hepatic tissue of spleens in animals without
portacaval shunt, the activities of the microsomal enzyme
Cytochrome c reductase and the cytosolic enzymes GPT and
GDH were only 14 - 30 % compared to normal liver.

Table 2 : Enzyme activities (U/g protein) in the homo-
          genate of the livers, normal spleen and
          "hepatized spleen".
          A = animals No.1-4; B = animals No. 5 and 6.

enzymes	liver A	B	spleen (normal)	liver tissue in the spleen A	B
Cyt.c-Red.	40± 6	55 ± 7	8 ± 3	12 ± 4	48 ± 11
GDH	178 ± 58	142 ± 52	3 ± 1	24 ± 8	106 ± 34
GPT	397 ± 91	720 ± 254	9 ± 4	74 ± 11	359 ± 34
GOT	263± 57	1190 ± 296	117 ± 24	223 ± 38	1236 ± 118
GLDH	220± 27	363 ± 100	36 ± 10	501 ± 82	1311 ± 105

The activity of GOT which is partially localized in the
mitochondria was 80 % of normal livers and GLDH, a true
mitochondrial enzyme, had an activity of 230 % of normal
livers. Thus portocaval shunt results in a 3-5 fold
increase of liver enzymes in the hepatized spleens.

Discussion

The results show that the activities of liver enzymes in
the spleen after liver cell transplantation depend on
their metabolic role and on a stimulation by the supply
of subtrates from portal blood. The portal blood reaches
the spleen in dilution from the general circulation via
spleenic artery.
Portal blood can stimulate the functions of the ectopic
liver. It has no influence of the proliferation rate and
growth of the transplanted hepatocytes (2).

References

1. Mito, M., Ebata, H., Kusano, M., Onishi, T., Saito, T.,
   Sakamoto, S. (1979). Morphology and function of isolated hepatocytes transplanted into rat spleen.
   Transplantation 28, 499 - 505
2. Mito, M., Ebata, H., Kusano, M., Onishi, T., Nozawa,M.
   (1981). Is potal venous blood essential for liver
   cell growth and proliferation ? Eur.Surg.Res.13, 57-58
3. Lösgen, H., Vonnahme, F.J., Stauch, D., Ohlendorf, S.,
   Schmidt, E., Brunner, G. (1984). Autologe Transplantation isolierter Leberzellen in die Milz bei der Ratte.
   In: Zelder, O. et al. (eds). Experimentelle und
   klinische Hepatologie IV; Schattauer, Stuttgart,
   pp 259-264

Reprints to:

Dr. med. H. Lösgen
Abt. Gastroenterologie und Hepatologie
Medizinische Hochschule Hannover

D - 3000 Hannover

22

The Immunogenicity of Isolated Liver Cells: Comparison of Complete Liver Cell Suspensions (LCS) versus Liver Parenchymal Cell Suspensions (LPS) in Two Different Allogeneic Inbred Rat Strain Combinations

R. ENGEMANN, H.-J. GASSEL, Th. SCHANG, A. THIEDE
and H. HAMELMANN

Abteilung für Allgemeinchirurgie, Christian-Albrechts-Universität Kiel

Zusammenfassung

Das Phänomen der Spontantoleranz nach orthotoper Rattenlebertransplantation ist beschrieben. Ziel der vorliegenden Untersuchung ist die Klärung der Frage, ob Injektion
gereinigter, class II antigenfreier Hepatozyten (LPS)
oder unseparierter Leberzellen (LCS) die Immunantwort des
Empfängers verändern. Die Ergebnisse der vollallogenen
BN - LEW Kombination werden denen der nur non-MHC inkompatiblen AS - LEW Kombination gegenübergestellt. Nach
i.V. Injektion der Zellen werden spenderspezifische Haut-
transplantate in beiden Kombinationen im normalen Intervall - verglichen mit den Kontrollgruppen - abgestoßen.
Nach Injektion der Zellen unter die Nierenkapsel und
anschließender histologischer Untersuchung zeigt sich,
daß in der vollallogenen BN - LEW Kombination LPS und LCS
nach 14 Tagen abgestoßen werden, in der AS - LEW Kombination werden Hepatozyten deutlich später abgestoßen als
die Zellen der LCS. Zur Toleranzinduktion ohne Immunsuppression scheint das intakte Gesamtorgan notwendig zu
sein. Die verzögerte Abstoßung der Hepatozyten nach Gabe
von LPS in der nur non-MHC inkompatiblen Kombination
beruht möglicherweise auf einer unterschiedlichen Antigen-
dichte (Antigenquantität) oder unterschiedlichen Antigen-

the method described by SEGLEN (SEGLEN, 1979). The viability of the cells was approx. 85 to 90 %.

Introduction

The phenomenon of spontaneous tolerance after orthotopic
liver transplantation in the rat model has been described
for the BN (RT1^n) - LEW (RT1^1) combination (ENGEMANN et
al., 1983, HOUSSIN et al., 1979). In contrast to this,
intraperitoneal injection of unseparated liver cells fails
to induce tolerance in the same strain combination
(GASSEL et al., 1984). The purpose of this study is to
determine whether injection of separated hepatocytes -
which clearly do not possess class II antigens - can
induce tolerance and whether there are differences
between the recipient's immune response to hepatocytes
(LPS) and that to liver cells (LCS) containing hepatocytes and other liver cells in the original ratio. Two
inbred rat strain combinations are compared. The fully
allogeneic BN - LEW combination, in which MHC and non-MHC
antigens are different, was used to investigate the
influence of class I and class II antigen differences on
the immune response. The AS - LEW combination served as a
weakly allogeneic system, in which only the non-MHC antigens are different. In this combination only the non-MHC
antigen differences should be able to affect the immune
response to LCS or LPS.

Material and Methods, Experimental Design

We used inbred rats of the strains BN and AS as donors,
LEW rats as recipients. DA and F344 rats served as third
party skin graft donors. Orthotopic liver transplantation
with rearterialization was performed as described in
detail elsewhere (ENGEMANN et al., 1985).
The liver cell suspensions were prepared in two steps:
(1). Liver cell disaggregation was performed by recirculating perfusion of the whole organ with collagenase buffer
(Collagenase type IV, Sigma GmbH, München) according to

mustern (Antigenqualität) der Hepatozyten und der Nicht-
hepatozyten in den injizierten Zellsuspensionen.

(2). To separate the LCS we used Percoll$^{(R)}$ density
gradient medium (Pharmacia Fine Chemicals, Freiburg). The
hepatocytes were resuspended in HEPES buffered RPMI 1640
medium. The cell viability was approx. 90 %, and the
number of nonparenchymal cells (marked by monoclonal antibodies O x 6 and W 3/25) was smaller than 1 %.
1 x 10^7 cells of LCS or LPS were injected i.v., or 1 x 10^6
cells were transplanted under the kidney capsule, to
examine the local alloreaction against the transplanted
cells. On day 14 or 30 after i.v. injection (subgroups
1 - 4) or subcapsular application (subgroups 5 - 8) donor-
specific and third party skin grafts were transplanted,
and the time of rejection was determined. The animals with
transplanted cells under their kidney capsule were
nephrectomized on day 14 or 30. p.i., and sections of the
kidneys were examined microscopically.

Results

A. Survival rates of liver allograft recipients and
rejection times of skin allografts
The long-term survival rate following orthotopic rat
liver transplantation was about 90 %. Donor-specific skin
allografts transplanted on day 20-30 post transplanta-
tionem were accepted for longer than 50 days.

Tables 1 and 2 show the rejection time of donor-specific
skin allografts following i.v. or subcapsular application
of LPS or LCS for the both combinations. Neither form of
application affected the rejection time of donor-specific
allografts, nor did the type of cell applied (LPS vs.
LCS). After each of these types of pretreatment with
liver cells skin grafts were rejected at normal intervals.
Third party skin grafts behaved similarly. In the combination AS - LEW, which is only non-MHC incompatible,
recipients of an AS liver allograft became long-term

Table 1: Rejection time of donor-specific skin allografts in the BN - LEW combination

Rejection time of donor specific skin allografts in the fully allogeneic
BN ⟶ LEW combination after application of LCS or LPS

group	celltype	injection mode	day of skin grafting after cell injection (d)	mean survival time of skin grafts (d)	number of animals
1	LPS	intravenous	+ 14	7,8 ± 1,2	8
2	LPS	intravenous	+ 30	7,6 ± 0,6	8
3	LCS	intravenous	+ 14	7,6 ± 0,6	8
4	LCS	intravenous	+ 30	7,9 ± 0,5	8
5	LPS	subcapsular	+ 14	7,5 ± 0,3	8
6	LPS	subcapsular	+ 30	7,8 ± 0,5	8
7	LCS	subcapsular	+ 14	7,4 ± 0,6	8
8	LCS	subcapsular	+ 30	7,5 ± 0,6	8
control				7,4 ± 0,6	15

Table 2: Rejection of donor-specific skin allografts in the AS - LEW combination

Rejection time of donor specific skin allografts in the non-MHC incompatible
AS ⟶ LEW combination after application of LCS or LPS

group	celltype	injection mode	day of skin grafting after cell injection (d)	mean survival time of skin grafts (d)	number of animals
1	LPS	intravenous	+ 14	9,5 ± 0,8	8
2	LPS	intravenous	+ 30	11,9 ± 1,1	8
3	LCS	intravenous	+ 14	10,4 ± 0,6	8
4	LCS	intravenous	+ 30	11,0 ± 0,6	8
5	LPS	subcapsular	+ 14	10,3 ± 1,1	8
6	LPS	subcapsular	+ 30	11,0 ± 0,9	8
7	LCS	subcapsular	+ 14	9,6 ± 0,6	8
8	LCS	subcapsular	+ 30	11,4 ± 0,7	8
control				10,0 ± 0,5	15

survivors and accepted donor-specific skin grafts. In
contrast, LPS or LCS that were applied i.v. or under the
kidney capsule did not induce skin graft acceptance, if
the skin was transplanted on day 14 or 30 after injection
of the cells. The skin grafts were rejected at normal
intervals compared to the control group. Third party skin
grafts were also rejected at normal intervals.

B. Histologic examinations

Following orthotopic rat liver transplantation with
rearterialization, 14 days after transplantation some
mononuclear infiltrations can be found in the periportal
area in both combinations. They costantly decrease in
long-term survivors (ENGEMANN et al., 1982).

Transplanted syngeneic hepatocytes could still be found
30 days after transplantation as a cell monolayer under
the morphologically unaltered kidney capsule (Fig. 1).

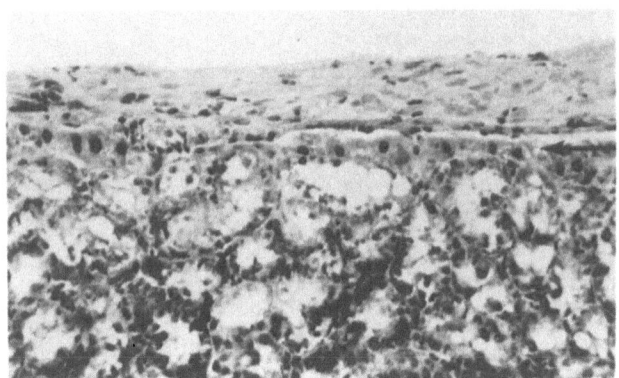

Figure 1: Syngeneic hepatocytes transplanted under the
          kidney capsule, 30 days after transplantation
          arrow shows hepatocytes.

In contrast, both LPS and LCS from a BN rat transplanted
under the kidney capsule of a LEW recipient were infiltrated by mononuclear cells after 14 days, as shown in
Figure 2. On day 30 after the injection no more LPS or
LCS could be seen. The capsule itself is thickened and
capillaries and mononuclear cells could be found (Fig. 3).

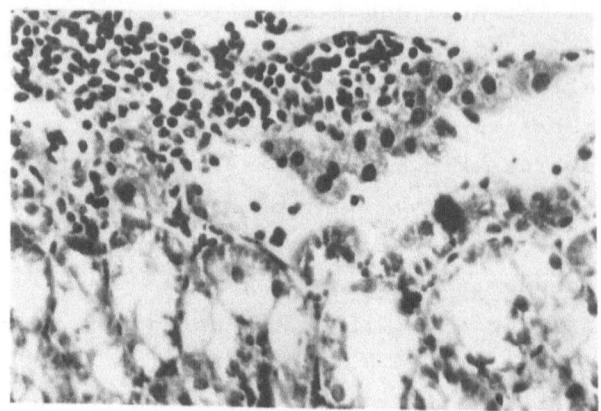

Figure 2: BN hepatocytes under the kidney capsule of
a LEW recipient, 14 days after injection of LPS

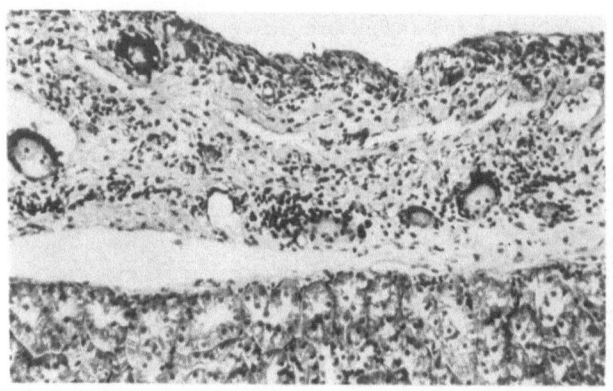

Figure 3: BN hepatocytes under the kidney capsule of
a LEW recipient, 30 days after injection of LPS

The histologic findings showed no difference between the
application of LPS and that of LCS.

The next two figures (Fig. 4, 5) show the alloreaction
against the LCS/LPS in the weakly allogeneic (only non-
MHC different) combination AS - LEW. In this group LCS
injected under the kidney capsule were infiltrated by
mononuclear cells on day 14 p.i., on day 30 p.i. hepatocytes could not be detected.

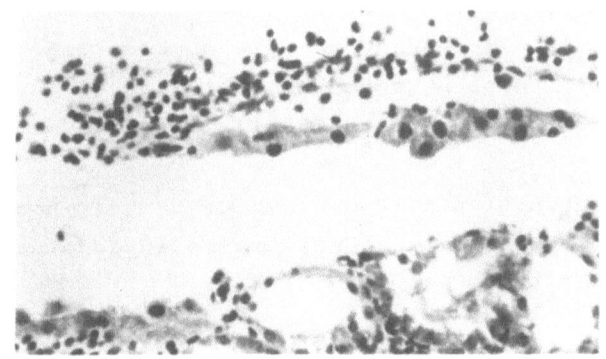

Figure 4: Weakly allogeneic AS hepatocytes under the kidney capsule of a LEW recipient 14 days **after injection of LCS**

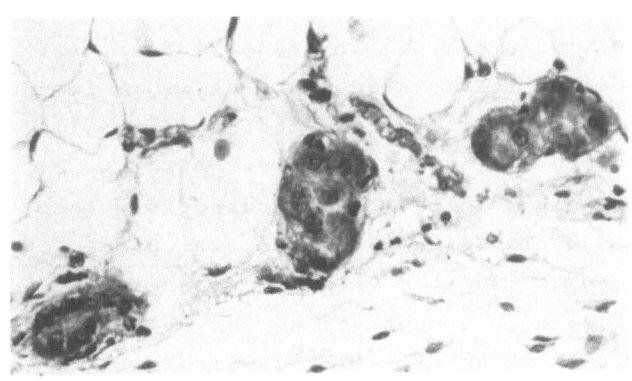

Figure 5: Weakly allogeneic hepatocytes under the kidney capsule of a LEW recipient 30 days after injection of LPS

After injection of LPS on day 30 p.i. groups of hepato-cytes showing unchanged morphology could be found in some sections.

The results can be summarized as follows:
1. In these two inbred rat strain combinations neither
   the i.v. injection of LPS or LCS nor the application
of the cells under the kidney capsule leads to tolerance
in the recipient, since donor-specific skin grafts transplanted 14 or 30 days after cell application are rejected

at normal intervals.

2. In the fully allogeneic BN - LEW combination no
difference can be seen in the alloreaction of the
recipients to the transplanted cells in our experimental
model.

3. In the combination AS - LEW, which is only non-MHC
incompatible, hepatocytes (LPS) are rejected clearly
later than LCS are.

Discussion

It is possible to enrich viable hepatocytes from the rat
liver by cell disaggregation and centrifugation in
Percoll$^{(R)}$ density gradient medium (SEGLEN 1979). LAUTEN-
SCHLAGER et al. (1983) showed that enzymatic disaggregation has no influence on the immunogenic potential of the
isolated cells. They stated that the major immunogenic
component of the rat liver is the Kupffer cells, which
strongly express class II antigens. BRENT et al. (1981)
described the possibility of inducing tolerance by
repeated injection of hepatocytes, which bear only class I
antigens, in combination with immunosuppressive drugs in
the mouse system. In contrast to the observations of
LAUTENSCHLAGER et al. (1981) regarding antigen expression
on hepatocytes, they state that hepatocytes possess a
normal complement of class I antigens. We also found hepatocytes that expressed class I antigens (own unpublished
data). This might be due to the collagenase treatment,
since antigen expression may change with changes in cell
function.

In contrast to Brent's observations, we showed that both
LCS and LPS transplanted under the kidney capsule in the
fully allogeneic combination BN - LEW are infiltrated by
mononuclear cells and rejected. Injection of hepatocytes
bearing only class I antigens failed to induce tolerance
in our model. We also did not detect any difference in
the rejection of skin grafts following injection of LPS,

bearing only class I antigens, or LCS, which bear class I
and class II antigens. Obviously the lack of Ia antigen
in LPS does not per se prevent the cells from being
rejected and does not lead to a state of immunologic
tolerance after cell injection. This was surprising,
since, with regard to orthotopic liver transplantation,
the BN - LEW combination is a low responder combination,
in which long-term acceptance of liver allografts occurs.
One would expect liver cell pretreatment to have at least
a slight effect on skin graft survival as well. However,
without immunosuppression the indicator system skin graft
may not be sensitive enough. Using the MHC compatible,
but non-MHC incompatible combination AS - LEW we clearly
demonstrate that not only the MHC coded genes induce an
immune response that leads to the destruction of the
liver cells under the kidney capsule within 14 days. LPS
are, however, rejected clearly later than LCS are. One
explanation for the difference between LPS and LCS with
regard to rejection could be that the density of non-MHC
antigens differs in LPS an other liver cells. The effect
would then be due to a different quantity of antigens on
the two cell populations. A second possibility would be a
qualitatively different antigen pattern of non-MHC antigens on hepatocytes and other liver cells which could
explain the morphologically different strength of the
immunologic attack. The latter point becomes very interes-
ting since we know that the expression of transplantation
antigens, e.g., Ia antigen, may be dependent on and vary
with the actual cell function. Combining these results
with those of former studies (GASSEL et al. 1984) we
conclude that for the induction of tolerance without
immunosuppression the orthotopic liver graft is
necessary. The observed tolerance is unlikely to be due
only to a "different" pattern of transplantation antigens
on liver cells.

References

1. Engemann, R., Ulrichs,K., Thiede,A., Müller-Ruchholtz, W., Hamelmann,H. (1983). A mechanism of tolerance in arterialized rat liver transplantation. Transplant. Proc. 15, 729 - 733

2. Houssin,D., Gigon,M., Franco,D., Szekely,A.M., Bismuth,H. (1979). Spontaneous long-term survival of liver allograft in inbred rats. Transplant. Proc.11, 567 - 570

3. Gassel,J., Engemann,R., Ulrichs,K., Müller-Ruchholtz, W., Thiede,A., Hamelmann,H. (1984). Toleranzinduktion durch Rattenlebertransplantation (ORLT). Vergleich von orthotoper Transplantation und Injektion von Leber- zellhomogenaten. In : O. Zelder, H.-D. Röher, M.Fischer, J.-Ch. Bode, Schattauer-Verlag Eds.: pp 251 - 254 Experimentelle und klinische Hepatologie

4. Engemann, R. (1985). The technique for orthotopic rat liver transplantation. In : Microsurgical Models in Rats for Transplantation Research. Ed.: Thiede,A., Deltz, E., Engemann, R., Springer Verlag (in press)

5. Seglen, P.O. (1979). Disaggregation and separation of rat liver cells. In : Cell Populations-Methodological Surveys-subseries (B): Biochemistry,Ed.: Eric Reid, Vol. 8

6. Engemann,R., Ulrichs,K., Thiede,A., Müller-Ruchholtz, W., Hamelmann, H. (1982). Value of a physiological liver transplant model in rats. Transplantation 33, 566 - 568

7. Lautenschlager, I., Nyman,N., Väänänen,V., Lehto,P., Virtanen,V., Häyry,P. (1983). Antigenic and Immunogenic Components in Rat Liver. Scand.J.Immunology 17, 61-83

8. Brent, L., Bain, A.G., Buttler,R., Horsburgh, T., Opara, S.C., Wood, P.J. (1981). The antigenicity of purified liver parenchymal cells. Transplant. Proc. 13, 860 - 862

9. Lautenschlager, I., Häyry, P. (1981). Expression of the major histocompatibility complex antigens on different liver cellular components in rat and man. Scand. J. Immunology 14, 421 - 426

Reprints to:

Dr. R. Engemann
Abteilung für Allgemeinchirurgie
Christian-Albrechts-Universität

D - 2300 Kiel

23
Membrane Expression of Autoantigens on Mechanically and Enzymatically Isolated Hepatocytes

G. GERKEN[1], M. MANNS[1], R. RAMADORI[1], T. PORALLA[1], H.P. DIENES[2] and K.H. MEYER ZUM BÜSCHENFELDE

[1]*I. Medizinische Klinik u.Poliklinik, Johannes-Gutenberg Universität Mainz, F.R.G.*
[2]*Institut für Pathologie, Johannes-Gutenberg, Universität Mainz, F.R.G.*

Zusammenfassung

Die Plasmamembranexpression von Leberzellmembran-Antigenen wurde mit indirekter Immunfluoreszenz (IF) und Immunelektronenmikroskopie (IELMI) an mechanisch und enzymatisch isolierten Kaninchenhepatozyten untersucht. 90 - 95 % der enzymatisch isolierten Hepatozyten, aber nur 40 - 60 % der mechanisch isolierten Hepatozyten waren intakt und vital. Eine Untergruppe der autoimmunen chronisch aktiven Hepatitis (CAH) weist zirkulierende Antikörper gegen ein mikrosomales Antigen aus Leber und Niere (LKM) auf. Die vermutete Membranexpression für LKM-Antigene konnte durch unsere Untersuchungen mit IF und IELMI an vitalen Kaninchenhepatozyten nicht nachgewiesen werden. Der als Referenzantikörper verwendete murine monoklonale Antikörper 2D3, der gegen eine organ- und speziesspezifische Determinante des leber-spezifischen Proteins (LSP) des Kaninchens gerichtet ist, reagierte mit der Membran vitaler, nicht aber mit der Membran vitaler Kaninchenhepatozyten. Dieser Antikörper eignet sich daher bei zukünftigen Untersuchungen als Marker für die Membranintegrität, d.h. der Vitalität von isolierten Kaninchenhepatozyten.

Introduction

Antigens expressed on the surface of the plasma membrane
of hepatocytes are candidate targets of immune reactions
responsible for liver cell destruction in inflammatory
liver diseases (8). Liver-kidney microsomal (LKM) autoantibodies directed against an antigen of the endoplasmic
reticulum characterize a subgroup of HBs-antigen negative
chronic active hepatitis (CAH) (11). LKM-antigen is
assumed to be expressed on the surface of the hepatocellular plasma membrane and it is therefore regarded as
a possible target antigen of immune reactions in liver
diseases (4), analogous to the microsomal antigen of the
thyroid in autoimmune thyroid diseases (3). Liver
specific lipoprotein (LSP) is an antigen complex containing organ-specific liver membrane expressed determinants.
Humoral and cellular immune reactions against this antigen fraction are found in inflammatory liver diseases of
various etiologies (8). Recently, a monoclonal antibody
against an organ- and species specific membrane expressed
determinant of rabbit LSP (2D3) was generated (9). In the
present study, the membrane expression of LKM-antigen and
of the organ-specific LSP determinant recognized by the
2D3 was investigated on hepatocytes isolated by a
mechanical and an enzymatical procedure. The membrane
expression of these antigens was evaluated by indirect
immunofluorescence (IF) and immunoelectronmicroscopy
(IELMI) and related to morphological criteria of viability and membrane integrity.

Materials and Methods

Four LKM-autoantibody positive sera from patients with
HBs-antigen negative CAH, two sera from patients with
primary biliary cirrhosis (PBC) positive for anti-mitochondrial antibodies (AMA), two sera from healthy blood
donors and their Ig G - fractions were included. Two
murine monoclonal antibodies generated against rabbit

LSP (9) were tested: 2D3 recognizing an organ- and species specific membrane determinant and 5B5 directed against a cytoplasmic determinant. Different isolation procedures of rabbit hepatocytes were performed. Mechanical isolation, described in detail elsewhere (2) is characterized by in vitro perfusion of excorporated rabbit liver. Enzymatical isolation technique was performed according to BERRY and FRIEND (1) modified by RAMADORI (10). Briefly, the rabbit liver was perfused in situ all the time and collagenase 0,05 % was added in the second perfusion step.

Control of hepatocyte integrity and viability was proved by light and phase-contrast microscopy and trypan blue exclusion test.

Results

Approximately 40 - 60 % of mechanically isolated hepato-cytes did not exhibit morphological criteria of plasma membrane integrity. The membrane of these cells was disrupted, irregularly shaped and desintegrated. Trypan blue was incorporated by these cells indicating cell necrosis and membrane desintegrity (Fig. 1a).

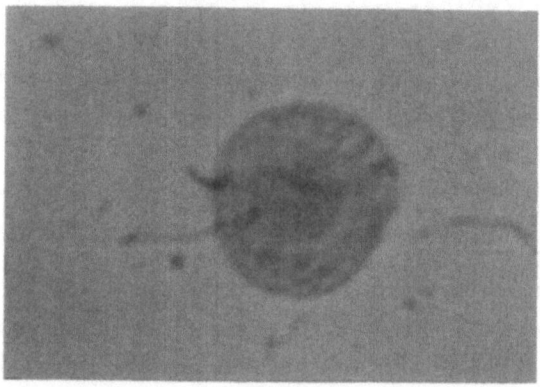

Fig. 1a: Mechanically isolated rabbit hepatocytes with disrupted and irregularly shaped membrane and inclusion of trypan blue (light- and phase-contrast microscopy, 250 x)

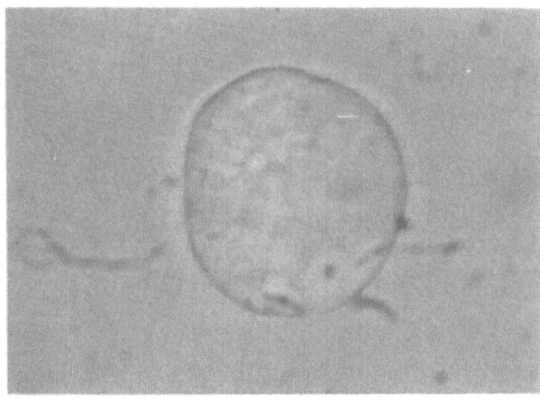

Fig. 1b: Enzymatically isolated rabbit hepatocytes with
         preserved membrane and exclusion of trypan blue
         (light- and phase-contrast microscopy, 250 x)

On the other hand, 90 - 95 % of enzymatically isolated
hepatocytes were intact and viable. The outline of these
cells was round and the plasma membrane was well-
preserved (Fig. 1b).

Examined by indirect IF, LKM-antibody positive sera and
their Ig G fractions did not stain the plasma membrane
of viable isolated hepatocytes (Fig. 2a).

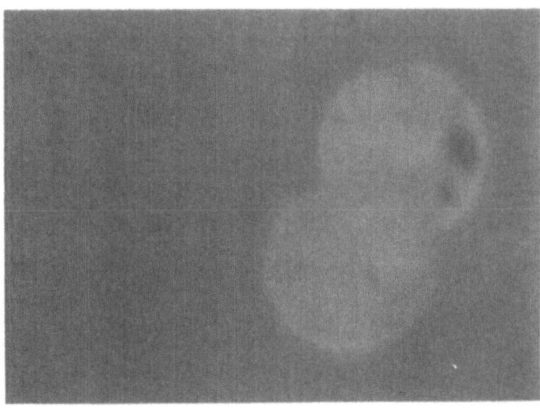

Fig. 2a: Lack of membrane binding of LKM-antibodies on
         enzymatically isolated viable hepatocytes
         (indirect IF, 250 x)

In contrast, a significant proportion of mechanically
isolated cells were stained by LKM positive sera (Fig.2b).

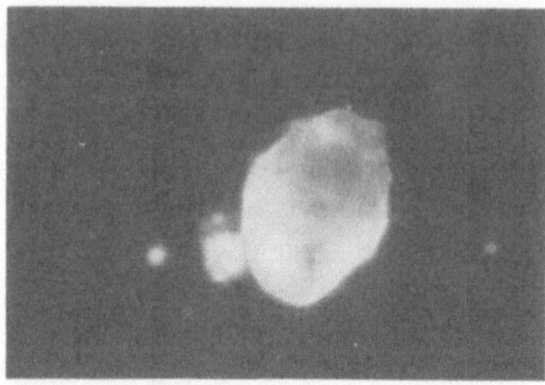

Fig. 2b: Staining pattern of LKM-antibodies on mechani-
         cally isolated non-viable rabbit hepatocytes
         (indirect IF, 250 x)

No membrane deposition of Ig G after incubation of viable
hepatocytes with LKM-positive sera and their IgG fractions was detected by IELMI (Fig. 2c). Submembranous
binding pattern was found when LKM positive sera were
tested on non-viable hepatocytes by IELMI (Fig. 2d).

On human liver tissue sections a reaction of LKM antibodies with the endoplasmic reticulum could be demonstrated by IELMI (Fig. 2e).

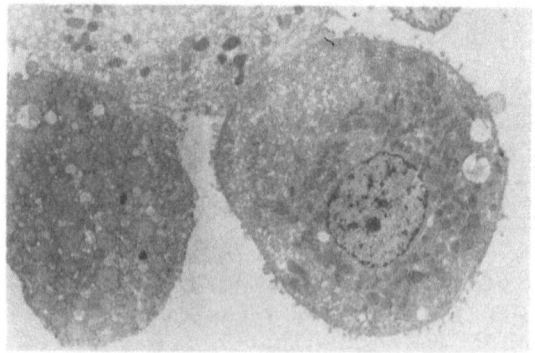

Fig. 2c: No membrane binding of LKM-antibodies to
         enzymatically isolated viable hepatocytes
         (IELMI, 3000 x)

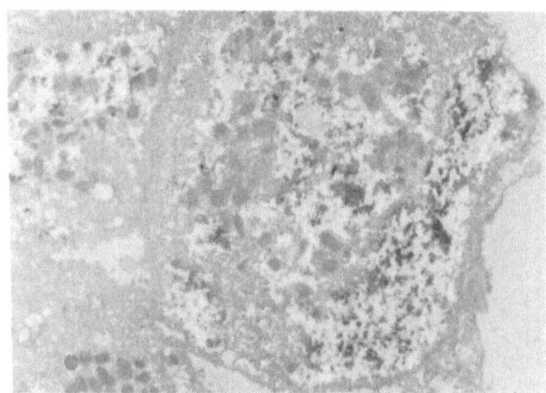

Fig. 2d: Reaction of LKM-antibodies with submembranous
structures of mechanically isolated non-viable
hepatocytes (IELMI, 3800 x)

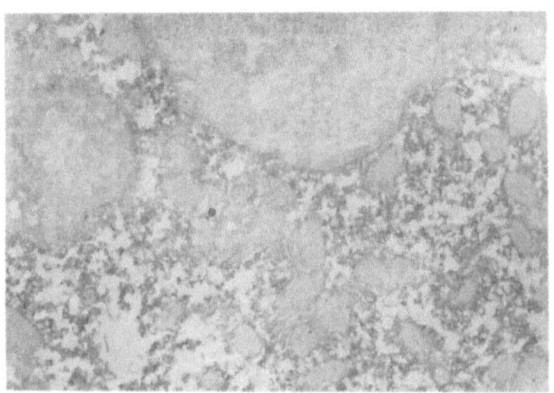

Fig. 2e: Localisation of LKM-antibody binding to the
endoplasmic reticulum of human liver tissue
sections (IELMI, 7800 x)

LKM and AMA positive sera and their IgG fractions were
absorbed with mechanically and enzymatically isolated
rabbit hepatocytes (6 x 10^6) and with purified rat liver
microsomes (Table 1). Absorbed samples and unabsorbed
controls were tested by IF on isolated hepatocytes and
on cryostat tissue sections of rat livers and kidneys.
In addition, LKM- RIA (7) and AMA-RIA for subtype M_2 (6)
were performed and correlated to IF. LKM antibodies were
not absorbed by viable isolated hepatocytes. In contrast,
LKM antibodies were absorbed by mechanically isolated
hepatocytes and by rat liver microsomes. AMA positive

Table 1: Results of absorption experiments of liver-kidney microsomal (LKM) and anti-mitochondrial antibodies (AMA) with mechanically and enzymatically isolated hepatocytes and with purified rat liver microsomes.

Sera absorbed with:	mechanically isolated hepato-cytes (6×10^6)			enzymatically isolated hepato-cytes (6×10^6)			rat liver microsomes (20 mg/µl)			unabsorbed test sera		
tested by :	IFT	RIA (LKM)	RIA (AMA-M_2)	IFT	RIA (AMA)	RIA (AMA-M_2)	IFT	RIA (LKM)	RIA (AMA-M_2)	IFT	RIA (LKM)	RIA (AMA-M_2)
LKM-sera (1:320) (n = 4)	–	–	–	+	+	–	–	–	–	+	+	–
LKM-IgG (1:320) (h = 4)	–	–	–	+	+	–	–	–	–	+	+	–
AMA-sera (1:320) (n = 2)	+	–	+	+	–	+	+	–	+	+	–	+
AMA-IgG (1:320) (n = 2)	+	–	+	+	–	+	+	–	+	+	–	+

IFT : indirect immunofluorescence test on rat liver and kidney tissue sections

RIA : radioimmunoassay for LKM antibodies and for subtype M_2 of AMA

n : number of different patient sera tested

sera were neither absorbed by non-viable or viable cells, nor by rat liver microsomes. IF and RIA coincided. These results provided evidence that LKM antigen is not expressed on the surface of viable hepatocytes.

The membrane expression of the LSP determinant recognized by 2D3 could be demonstrated on intact and viable hepato-cytes (Fig. 3a). In contrast, 2D3 did not react with disrupted hepatocytes (Fig. 3b). The plasma membrane expression of the LSP determinant recognized by 2D3 was also demonstrated by IELMI on viable isolated cells (Fig. 3c).

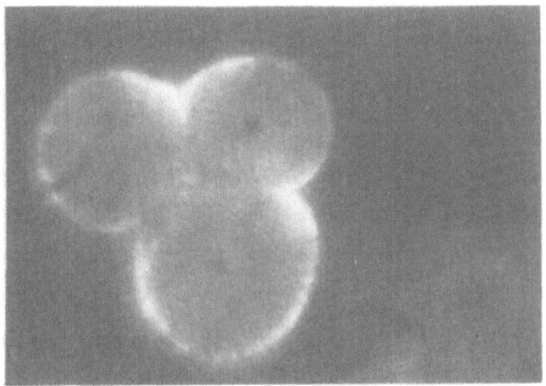

Fig. 3a: Linear membranous deposition of murine mono-
         clonal antibody 2D3 on enzymatically isolated
         viable hepatocytes (ind. IF, 250 x)

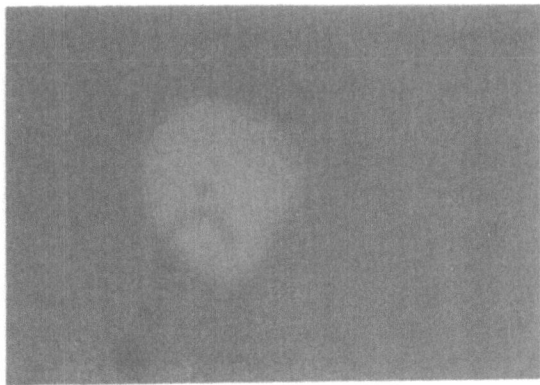

Fig. 3b: Lack of membrane binding of 2D3 on mechanically
         isolated non-viable rabbit hepatocytes
         (indirect IF, 250 x)

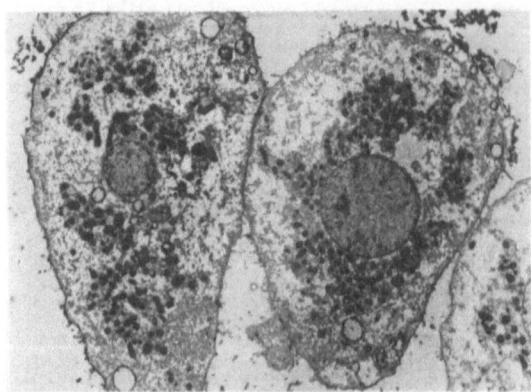

Fig. 3c: Linear membrane binding of 2D3 on viable rabbit
         hepatocytes (IELMI, 3800 x)

Discussion

The data presented give no evidence for a plasma membrane
expression of LKM-antigen on viable isolated rabbit
hepatocytes. This observation is in contrast to data
recently published (4), describing a membrane expression
of LKM-antigen on enzymatically isolated hepatocytes. We
suggest that the assumed membrane expression of the antigen was due to hepatocytes with desintegrated plasma
membranes which allowed a penetration of the LKM-auto-
antibodies to submembranous parts of the endoplasmic
reticulum. By indirect IF and IELMI on non-viable hepatocytes we succeeded in demonstrating the reaction of LKM
autoantibodies with the endoplasmic reticulum. However,
the expression of LKM-antigen on the liver cell surface
due to pathological conditions leading to LKM autoantibody positive CAH has to be considered. The potential
membrane expression of antigens may be evoked by etiological agents of liver diseases as has been demonstrated in
halothane hepatitis (5) and alcohol induced liver disease
(12). So far, methodological difficulties may hamper to
prove this hypothesis. Firstly, the etiological agent of
LKM-antibody positive CAH is unknown and thus similar
experiments as performed in halothane hepatitis and
alcoholic liver disease cannot be done in experimental
animals. Secondly, it seems difficult to isolate viable

human hepatocytes from biopsies of patients with LKM-antibody positive CAH to investigate the membrane expression of LKM-antigen. The potential need of viable hepatocytes with intact plasma membranes to demonstrate the membrane expression of an antigen is evidenced by the monoclonal antibody 2D3. The plasma membrane expression of the LSP determinant recognized by 2D3 was demonstrable only on viable enzymatically isolated hepatocytes with complete membrane integrity.

Finally, the monoclonal antibody 2D3 can be used in future studies as a marker for cell surface integrity and viability of isolated or cultured hepatocytes. It can also be applied in blocking experiments to evaluate whether this LSP-determinant is a target of humoral or cellular immune reactions in hepatitis.

Acknowledgements

We are indebted to Miss U. Dang for exellent technical assistance. This work was supported by Deutsche Forschungsgemeinschaft, grant Ma 938/1-1 and grant Ra 362/1-1.

References

1. Berry, N.M., Friend, D.S.(1969). High-vield preparation of isolated rat liver parenchymal cells. A biochemical and fine structural study. J.Cell.Biol. **43**, 506

2. Hopf, U., Meyer zum Büschenfelde, K.H., Arnold, W. (1976). Detection of a liver-membrane autoantibody in HBs-Ag negative chronic active hepatitis. N. Engl.J.Med. **294**, 578

3. Khoury, E.L., Hammond,L., Bottazzo, G.F., Doniach, D. (1981). Presence of the organ-specific microsomal auto-antigen in the surface of human thyroid cells in culture: its involvement in complement-mediated cyto-toxicity. Clin.exp. Immunol. **45**, 316

4. Lenzi, M., Bianchi,F.B., Casani,F., Pisi,E. (1984). Liver cell surface expression of the antigen reacting

with liver-kidney microsomal antibody (LKM).
Clin.exp. Immunol. 55, 36

5. MacSween,R.N.M., Burt,A., Anthony, R.S., Hislop, W.S.
(1980). Liver membrane antibodies in alcoholic liver
disease (Abstract). Gastroenterology 79, 1114

6. Manns,M., Meyer zum Büschenfelde,K.H. (1982). A mitochondrial antigen-antibody system in cholestatic liver
disease detected by radioimmunoassay. Hepatology 2, 1

7. Manns,M., Meyer zum Büschenfelde,K.H., Slusarczyk,J.,
Dienes,H.P. (1984). Detection of liver-kidney microsomal autoantibodies by radioimmunoassay and their
relation to antimitochondrial antibodies in inflammatory liver diseases. Clin.exp.Immunol. 57, 600

8. Meyer zum Büschenfelde, K.H., Manns, M. (1984).
Mechanisms of autoimmune liver disease.
Sem. Liver Dis. 4, 1, 26

9. Poralla, T., Dippold,W., Dienes,H.P., Manns,M.,
Meyer zum Büschenfelde,K.H. (1984). A monoclonal antibody directed against an organ-specific liver cell
membrane antigen in rabbits. J.Immunol.Meth.68, 341

10.Ramadori,G., Lenzi,M., Dienes,H.P., Meyer zum Büschenfelde, K.H. (1983). Binding properties of mechanically and enzymatically isolated hepatocytes for IgG
and C_3. Liver 3, 358

11.Rizzetto, M., Swana,G., Doniach,D. (1973). Microsomal
antibodies in active chronic hepatitis and other
disorders. Clin.exp.Immunol. 15, 331

12.Vergani,D., Mieli-Vergani,G., Alberti,A., Neuberger,J.,
Eddlestone,A.L.W.F., Davis,M., Williams,R. (1980).
Antibodies to the surface of halothane altered rabbit
hepatocytes in patients with severe halothane-
associated hepatitis. N.Engl.J.Med. 303, 66

Reprints to:

Prof.Dr.Dr. K.H. Meyer zum Büschenfelde
Leiter der I.Medizinischen Klinik und Poliklinik
der Johannes-Gutenberg Universität Mainz
Langenbeckstr. 1   D - 6500 Mainz   (FRG)

24

Inhibition of Collagen Biosynthesis in Cultured Mesenchymal Cells of Human Liver by Malotilate: Treatment of Patients with Chronic Active Liver Diseases – First Results

M. SCHNEIDER, B. HÖGEMANN, J. RAUTERBERG*, G. POTT
and U. GERLACH

*Medical Clinic and Policlinic of the University of Münster, Division of Gastroenterology,
Institute of Arteriosclerosis Research of the University of Münster, F.R.G.

Zusammenfassung

Nach Untersuchungen an CCL_4- und TAA-geschädigten Ratten-lebern inhibiert Malotilate die Bindegewebsneubildung. Zellkulturversuche an "smooth muscle cell-like" Zellen menschlicher Leber und an embryonalen Lungenfibroblasten zeigen eine dosisabhängige Hemmung der Kollagenbiosynthese. Gemessen im Kulturmedium, ist die Gesamtprotein-synthese in etwas geringerem Maß als die Kollagensynthese reduziert. Die Medium P-III-P-Konzentration fällt unter Malotilate ebenfalls ab. Erste Behandlungsergebnisse von Patienten mit chronisch aktiven Lebererkrankungen unter-schiedlicher Genese zeigen einen deutlichen Abfall der Serumkonzentrationen für GOT und GPT sowie für P-III-P.

Introduction

Hepatic fibrosis is characterized by an increased deposi-tion of fibrous connective tissue. Activity of collagen synthesis is enhanced during fibroplasia, reflected by an elevated procollagen-III-peptide (P-III-P) concentra-tion in serum of patients with chronic active liver diseases (1). Standard therapy in chronic active liver diseases is antiinflammatory and immunsuppressive. Drugs inhibiting synthesis of connective tissue components may give a more causal therapy of these diseases.

179

Malotilate (diisopropyl 1,3-dithiol 2-ylidene-malonate) protects rats from liver injury induced by carbon tetrachloride (CCL_4), dimethylnitrosamine and thioacetamide (TAA), enhances protein synthesis and cell proliferation in cultured rat hepatocytes and reduces collagen synthesis in CCL_4-induced chronic hepatitis in rats (2, 3).

This contribution is designed to summarize the influence of malotilate on collagen biosynthesis in cells grown from explants of human fibrotic liver ("smooth muscle cell like cells") (4) of human liver and of embryonary lung fibroblasts and to give first results from patients with chronic active liver diseases treated with malotilate.

Material and Methods

Cells were cultivated in 15 ml Eagle's medium, Dulbecco's modification (Behringwerke Marburg, Germany), containing 10 % (v/v) fetal bovine serum and ascorbic acid (50 µg/ml). Malotilate was added in different concentrations (from 5 to 500 µg/ml) to each medium, and P-III-P was measured at 10 min., 30 min., 2 h, 6 h and 24 h in the medium by RIA (Hoechst, Frankfurt, Germany). After 24 h the medium was changed to serum-free and glycine-free medium, with 2,5 µCi/ml ^{14}C-glycine and 2,5 µCi/ml ^{14}C-proline (Amersham Corp., Munich, Germany) added and with the same malotilate concentration as in the first 24 h. Total protein and collagen in the medium were determined after 48 h incubation with malotilate as described (5).

Results and Discussion

The effect of malotilate on collagen and protein synthesis showed no difference between the two cell types. Malotilate led to a dose-dependent decrease in collagen and, to a somewhat lesser extent, in total protein synthesis the main slope occurring between malotilate concentrations from 20 µg/ml to 50 µg/ml (Fig. 1).

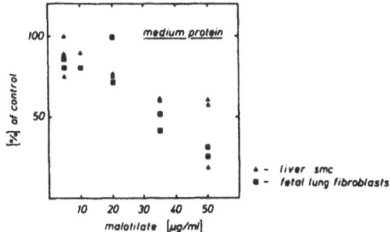

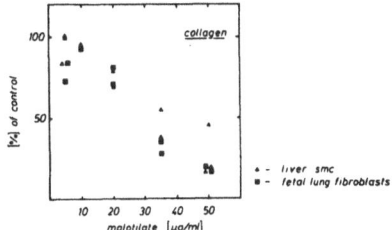

Figure 1

Gelelectrophoresis and fluorography of medium proteins
after incubation with malotilate showed a relatively
stronger inhibition of procollagen chains than of
fibronectin.

Additionally, procollagen-III-peptide concentration in
the culture medium was followed during the first 24 hours
after malotilate addition. In general the initial concentration of P-III-P which was due to the presence of fetal
serum in the medium did not increase during incubation.
In the medium of SMCL cell cultures there was even a
decrease between 30 min and 6 h, which was more pronounced in the malotilate-treated cells than in controls
(Fig. 2). Similar results have been obtained with
embryonal fibroblasts (Fig. 3).

Treated and untreated cells were investigated morphologically by light- and electron microscopy. Cells cultivated in medium containing fetal bovine serum demonstrated
no difference from cells incubated for 24 hours in serum-
free medium. Malotilate-treated cells seem to be of small
extension, and more multinuclear cells were found. By
electron microscope, lipid drops and enlarged mitochondria were seen in contrast to untreated cells.

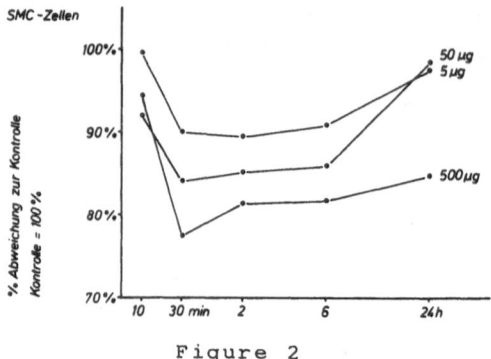

Figure 2

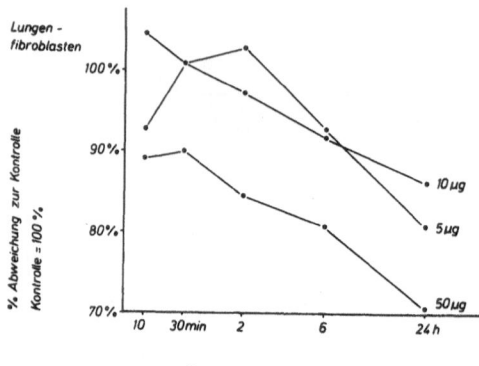

Figure 3

In a phase 2 uncontrolled clinical study we have treated
14 patients with chronic active hepatitis, chronic
alcoholic hepatitis, primary sclerosing cholangitis and
primary biliary cirrhosis. Before treatment with malotilate, dose 1500 mg/day, patients had been untreated for
at least two months. Malotilate was given for 4 - 6 months.
After 4-8 weeks, aminotransferase were reduced by half in
all patients; marked decreases in serum P-III-P concentrations were noted after 4 - 6 months. Histological
investigations in some patients showed a decrease in the
estimated degree of fibrosis and a reduction in single
cell necrosis.

In conclusion, results from cultivated mesenchymal human
cells show a dose-dependent inhibition of collagen biosynthesis by malotilate, although the mechanism is not
yet known. The therapeutical effect on patients with

chronic active liver diseases observed in an uncontrolled clinical study must be examined by controlled studies of a greater number of patients.

References

1. Rhode,H., Vargas,L., Hahn,E., Kalbfleisch, H., Bruguera, M., Timpl,R. (1979). Radioimmunoassay for type III procollagen peptide and its application to human disease. European Journal of Clinical Investigation 9, 451 - 459

2. Monna,T. (1982). Effects of malotilate on experimental cirrhosis induced by carbon tetrachloride (CCL_4) or egg yolk sensitization. Malotilate symposium, Stockholm, Abstracts

3. Guillouzo, A., Clément,B., Latinier,M.F., Brissot,P., Dumont, J.-M. (1984). Effects of malotilate on human and rat hepatocytes in pure and mixed culture. Malotilate symposium, Berne, Abstracts

4. Voss,B., Rauterberg,J., Pott,G., Brehmer,U., Allam,S., Lehmann,R., Bassewitz, D.v. (1982). Nonparenchymal cells cultivated from explants of fibrotic liver resemble endothelial and smooth muscle cells from blood vessel walls. Hepatology 2, 18 - 28

5. Rauterberg,J., Allam,S., Brehmer, U., Wirth, W., Hauss, W.-H. (1977). Characterization of the collagen synthesized by cultured human smooth muscle cells from fetal and adult aorta. Hoppe-Seyler's Z.Physiol. Chem. 358, 401 - 407

Reprints to:

Dr. med. M. Schneider
Westfälische Wilhelms-Universität
Abteilung Innere Medizin B
Albert-Schweitzer-Str. 35

D - 4400 Münster

25
Lack of Hormonal Response in Liver Cells from Rats with Extrahepatic Cholestasis*

J. SCHÖLMERICH, M.-S. BECHER, U. BAUMGARTNER and W. GEROK

Department of Internal Medicine, University of Freiburg

Zusammenfassung

Gallensäuren verändern Membranen und führen in vitro zu
einem Verlust der Hormonantwort. Die glukoneogenetische
Kapazität isolierter Leberzellen von Ratten mit extra-
hepatischer Cholestase und deren hormonelle Kontrolle
wurde untersucht. Während Zellen scheinoperierter Tiere
in Gegenwart von Glucagon einen Anstieg der Glukosefrei-
setzung von 63 % aufwiesen, reagierten Zellen von
Cholestasetieren nicht. Da andere metabolische Reaktionen
erhalten waren, folgern wir, daß ein Verlust der hormo-
nellen Kontrolle in der Leber an Störungen der Glukose-
homeostase bei cholestatischen Erkrankungen beteiligt sein
könnte.

Bile salts (BS) reduce the susceptibility of isolated rat
liver cells to peptide hormones in vitro (1). This effect
may be due to alterations of membrane fluidity and
destruction of submembraneous structures by BS which have
been described in several models (2). It is, however,
unknown if this loss of hormonal control has a role in

---

* Footnote: This work was supported by the Deutsche
            Forschungsgemeinschaft (SFB 154: Klinische und
            experimentelle Hepatologie, Freiburg)

cholestasis in vivo. In order to elucidate a possible
alteration of hormone response in cholestasis, we studied
isolated cells from rats 1 - 6 days after ligation of the
common bile duct regarding their response to glucagon
using gluconeogenesis as parameter. In addition, several
parameters of cell function and membrane leakage were
studied.

Materials and Methods

Materials: Female Sprague-Dawley rats (weight 239 ± 35 g)
were used. All biochemicals and chemicals used for buffers
and media were obtained in analytical purity. Glucagon
was from Serva (Heidelberg, West Germany).

Methods: Cholestasis: After an overnight fast the common
bile duct was ligated atraumatically after median laparotomy. Sham-operated controls were treated identically
with the exception that the ligature was not tightened.
Isolation and incubation of cells: After 24 h fasting
isolation of cells, viability testing, cell counting and
incubation were essentially done as described previously
(1). Three different groups of three incubations each
done with cells from each animals in Krebs-Ringer-
Bicarbonate buffer (pH 7.4, $37^{\circ}C$, gassed with Carbogen)
for 1 hour: Either alanine (10 mM) alone; or alanine
(10 mM), lactate (5.5 mM), and pyruvate (1.1 mM); or
alanine (10 mM) and glucagon (1 µM) were added from the
beginning to the incubation medium. Incubation was
stopped after 1 hour by rapid centrifugation (30 xg,
1 min) at $4^{\circ}C$. Supernatants and pellets were collected
and used for analysis (3).

Results

A similar weight decrease occured in both groups of rats.
The yield of viable cells isolated from the liver of
cholestatic rats decreased with duration of cholestasis
and was always lower than that obtained from shamoperated

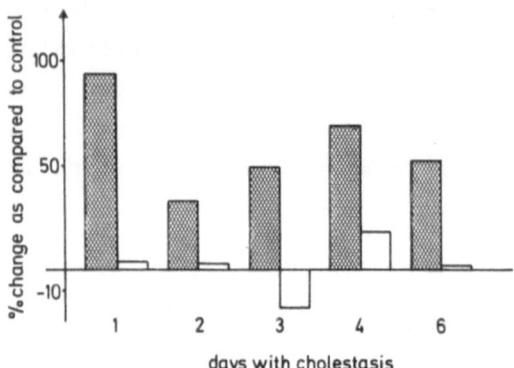

Figure 1: Percent increase of glucose release in the
           presence of alanine (10 mM), lactate (5.5 mM),
           and pyruvate (1,1 mM)   (▨▨▨▨), or alanine
           (10 mM) and glucagon (1 µM) (☐), as compa-
           red to incubations with alanine only. Each bar
           gives the difference as percent between the
           means of three incubations of cells from
           cholestatic rats. Modified from 5.

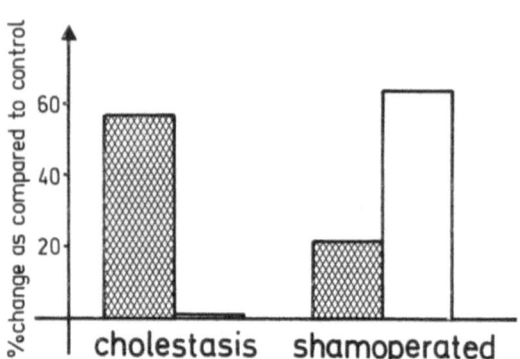

Figure 2: Percent increase of glucose release in the
           presence of alanine (10 mM), lactate (5.5 mM),
           and pyruvate (1.1 mM)   (▨▨▨▨), or alananine
           (10 mM) and glucagon (1 µM) (☐). Each bar
           represents the difference as percent between
           the means of 18 (cholestasis) or 6 (sham-
           operated) incubations. Modified from 5.

controls. The average lactate/pyruvate ratio in the
incubation medium was not different between both groups.
Lactate and pyruvate addition to the incubation medium
resulted in an increase of glucose release of 56 % in
cells from cholestatic animals and of 22 % in controls
while basic glucose release was lower in the cholestatic
than in the shamoperated group (C: 3.0 $\pm$ 0.7 μmoles/10^6
cells/h; S: 4.1 $\pm$ 1.5).

Glucagon addition did never result in an increase of
glucose release in cells from cholestatic livers regardless of the duration of cholestasis (figure 1). In
contrast, cells from shamoperated rats showed a 63 %
increase (figure 2).

Discussion

Stimulation of gluconeogenesis is preserved in viable
isolated liver cells from fasted rats (4). Concentration
or affinity of membrane receptors can be modified by
alterations of membrane fluidity which, furthermore, is
changed by BS (2). Accordingly it has been shown that BS
alter hormone-receptor interaction, thus leading to a loss
of hormonal control in isolated liver cells from normal
rats in the presence of pathological BS concentrations (1).
The data presented in this study suggest that this loss
occurs also in cells from cholestatic livers,i.e.in vivo.
Since the metabolic response to substrate supply is preserved we do not believe that intrinsic metabolic impair-
ments are the reason for the missing hormonal response.
This impairment of hormonal control in cholestatic livers
may have a role in the disturbance of the metabolism of
glucose and other substrates in cholestatic conditions.

References

1) Schölmerich, J., Becher,M.-S., Schmidt,K., Schubert,R.,
   Kremer, B., Feldhaus, S., Gerok, W. (1984).
   Hepatology 4, 661 - 666

2) Olson, J.R., Hosko, M.J., Fujimoto, J.M. (1979)
   Life Sci. 25, 2043 - 2050

3) Bergmeyer, H.U. (1974). Methoden der enzymatischen
   Analyse, Verlag Chemie Weinheim

4) Sies, E.A., Wieland, O.H. (1975) Biochem. Biophys.
   Res. Commun. 64, 323 - 330

5) Schölmerich, J., Becher,M.-S., Baumgartner, U.,
   Gerok, W. Biochem. Biophys. Res. Commun. in press

Reprints to:

Dr. J. Schölmerich
Medizinische Universitätsklinik

D - 7800 Freiburg
West Germany

26

Regulation of the Glucose/Glucose-6-Phosphate Cycle in Cultured Hepatocytes by Insulin and Glucagon

B. CHRIST, I. PROBST and K. JUNGERMANN

Institut für Biochemie, Georg-August-Universität, Göttingen

Zusammenfassung

Die Regulation des Glucose/Glucose-6-Phosphat-Zyklus durch Insulin und Glucagon wurde in Leberzellen in Primärkultur untersucht. Zur Abschätzung der Fluxraten des Zyklus wurde einerseits der Verbrauch von $(U^{14}C, 2^{3}H)$-Glucose, andererseits der Verbrauch von $(2^{3}H)$-Glucose, die Bildung von $(U^{14}C)$-Glucose aus $(U^{14}C)$-Glykogen bestimmt.

Unter dem Einfluß von Insulin war eine weitgehende Hemmung des Fluxes von Glucose-6-Phosphat zu Glucose durch die Glucose-6-Phosphatase bei gleichzeitigem Anstieg des Fluxes von Glucose zu Glucose-6-Phosphat durch die Glucokinase zu beobachten. Glucagon zeigte keinen Einfluß auf den Glucoseverbrauch in der Glucokinase Reaktion. Es war aber ein starker Anstieg der Glucose-Bildung aus Glykogen durch die Glucose-6-Phosphatase Reaktion zu verzeichnen. Zusammenfassend ergab sich bei Insulinbehandlung der Leberzellen eine Zunahme des Netto-Fluxes von Glucose zu Glucose-6-Phosphat von 200 % - 365 %, wohingegen Glucagon die Glucose-Bildung aus Glykogen um 500 % stimulierte. Ob Insulin und Glucagon die Aktivität der Zyklusenzyme Glucose-6-Phosphatase und Glucokinase direkt oder indirekt steuert, kann aus den vorliegenden Versuchen nicht abgeleitet werden.

Introduction

Glucose homoeostasis of the organism is maintained
primarily by the liver, which takes up glucose for
glycogen synthesis and glycolysis in the absorptive
phase and liberates glucose, when needed via glycogenolysis and gluconeogenesis. The glucostat function of the
liver is mainly under control of the glucoregulatory
hormones insulin and glucagon, the former increasing
glucose uptake, the latter enhancing glucose output. The
decisive parameter for net uptake or release of glucose
by the liver is the net flux at the glucose/glucose-6-
phosphate cycle. It was therefore the intention of the
present work, to investigate the regulation of the cycle
by insulin and glucagon in hepatocyte cultures.

Methods

Hepatocytes were maintained in primary culture for 48 h
with medium 199 containing 5 mM glucose, 10 nM insulin
and 100 nM dexamethasone (1). The short-term effect of
insulin and glucagon (100 nM) on glucose flow at the
glucose/glucose-6-phosphate cycle was studied during the
period from 48 h - 52 h.
If glucose was the only exogenous substrate, it was uniformly labelled with ^{14}C and in position 2 with ^{3}H
(Fig. 1).

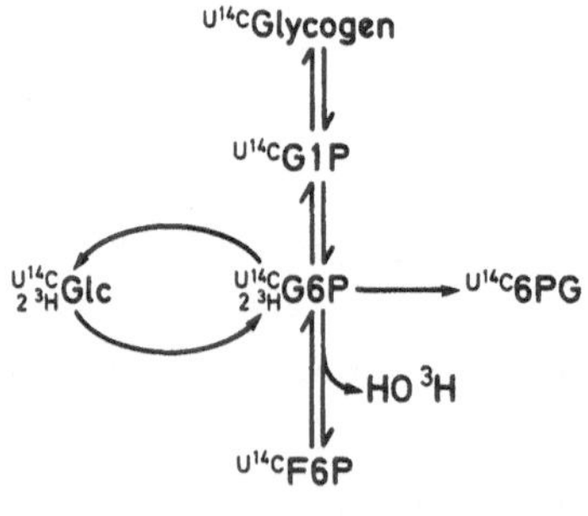

Fig. 1: Flow radiolabel at the glucose/glucose-6-phosphate
cycle. Glc = glucose, G6P (G1P) = glucose-6 (1)-
phosphate, 6PG = 6-phosphogluconate, F6P =
fructose-6-phosphate.

The parameters measured were the utilization of ^{3}H- and
^{14}C-glucose and the generation of tritated water (Fig. 2A)
(If glucose-6-phosphate totally equilibrates with
fructose-6-phosphate, the generation of HO^{3}H equals the
utilization of ^{3}H-glucose). ^{3}H-glucose utilization can be
regarded as minimal flux through glucokinase (GK), the
difference of ^{3}H- and ^{14}C-glucose utilization as the
minimal reverse flux through glucose-6-phosphatase
(G6Pase), and the utilization of ^{14}C-glucose as the net
flow at the cycle (Fig. 2 B).

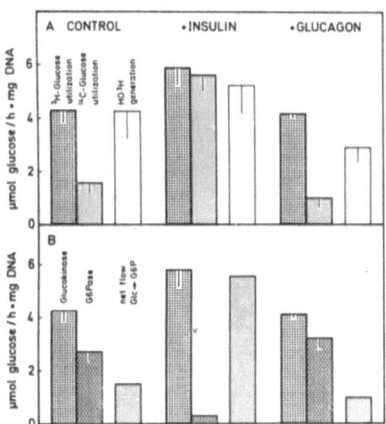

Fig. 2: Effects of insulin and glucagon on (A) the
        utilization of 2^{3}H - and U^{14}C-glucose and the
        generation of tritiated water and on (B) flux
        through glucokinase, reverse flux through glucose-
        6-phosphatase (G6Pase) and net flow of glucose
        label at the glucose/glucose-6-phosphate cycle
        in cultured hepatocytes.

Starting with labelled glucose the reverse flux of
glucose-6-phosphate to glucose via G6Pase can never
exceed the forward flux from glucose to glucose-6-phos-
phate via GK; thus only net glucose uptake but not glucose
release can be measured by the above described technique.
Therefore glycogen was ^{14}C-labelled by growing the
hepatocytes with U^{14}C-glucose from 24 h - 48 h (2). The
short-term effect of the hormones was then studied from
48 h - 52 h in the presence of 2^{3}H-glucose and U^{14}C-

glucose-6-phosphate generated from glycogen. The utilization of 2^3H-glucose represents the minimal flux through
GK and the generation of U^{14}C-glucose the reverse flux
through G6Pase via glycogenolysis but not via gluconeogenesis (Fig. 3). Net glucose release can only be observed
under these conditions if glucose formation from glycogen
exceeds glucose uptake. Radioactive glucose and tritiated
water were separated by ion exchange chromatography using
Dowex borate and formate as exchange matrix.

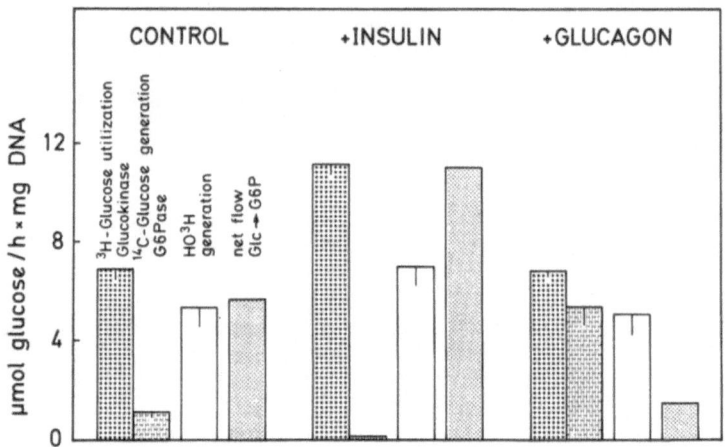

Fig. 3: Effects of insulin and glucagon on the utiliza-
        tion of 2^3H-glucose = flux through glucokinase,
        on the formation of U^{14}C-glucose from U^{14}C-
        glycogen = flux through glucose-6-phosphatase,
        on formation of tritiated water and on net flow
        of label at the glucose/glucose-6-phosphate
        cycle in cultured hepatocytes.

Results

The utilization of glucose via the glycolytic pathway is
regulated by insulin and glucagon. Insulin stimulated
lactate formation from glucose (μmol C_6 unit/h x mg DNA)
from 1.4 to 4.0, whereas glucagon suppressed it to 4.0
(1). Moreover, insulin stimulated the minimal flux through
glucokinase (GK) to 140 % whereas the reverse flux through
glucose-6-phosphatase (G6Pase) was reduced to 10 %

(Fig. 2 B). Glucagon did not influence glucose flux
through GK but only slightly increased the flux through
G6Pase to 120 % (Fig. 2 B). Under these experimental
conditions the net flow of glucose to glucose-6-phosphate
was markedly increased by insulin to 365 %, while it was
decreased by glucagon to 60 % (Fig. 2 B).

Starting with $U^{14}C$, 2^3H-glucose no net glucose output can
be observed, of course, since the reverse flow through
G6Pase cannot surpass the forward flow through GK. Only
with simultaneous labelling of glucose and glucose-6-
phosphate a net formation of glucose at the glucose/
glucose-6-phosphate cycle can be observed. Using $U^{14}C$-
glycogen as a source of $U^{14}C$-glucose-6-phosphate together
with 2^3H-glucose it was found that insulin caused a
pronounced stimulation to 165 % of glucose flux through
GK, whereas formation of glucose via G6Pase was totally
depressed (Fig. 3). Consequently insulin increased the
net flow of glucose label to glucose-6-phosphate to
nearly 200 %. Conversely, glucagon had no effect on
glucose flux through GK, but stimulated glucose flux
through G6Pase to 500 %. In turn, net flow of glucose
label to glucose-6-phosphate was diminished to 25 % under
the influence of glucagon (Fig. 3). Since glucose-6-
phosphate was labelled only from glycogen and not, in
addition, from pyruvate, the net flow at the cycle was
underestimated; net glucose release could not be observed.

Discussion

The present study has shown that insulin strongly inhibited and that glucagon increased flux through glucose-6-
phosphatase (G6Pase), and, moreover, that insulin enhanced
flux through glucokinase (GK). The hormones may influence
directly the activity of the enzymes G6Pase and GK or
they may act indirectly at other key regulatory enzymes
of carbohydrate metabolism. The present experiments do
not allow to distinguish between a direct or indirect

mode of hormone action. A direct hormone effect on G6Pase
might be indicated by the findings that preincubation of
rat liver microsomes with insulin or glucagon led to a
25 % inhibition or 50 % activation, respectively, of the
enzyme activity (3) and that a low molecular weight
factor from insulin treated plasma membranes, the puta-
tive insulin mediator, suppressed the enzyme activity in
microsomes by 40 % (4). These in vitro effects in micro-
some preparations were much smaller than the in vivo
effects in cultured hepatocytes seen in this investigation.
A possible direct hormonal regulation of glucose-6-phos-
phatase would be of prime physiological significance;
the problem is presently under investigation using the
model of cultured hepatocytes.

References

1. Probst, I., Schwartz, P. and Jungermann,K. (1982).
   Eur.J.Biochem. 126,   271 - 278
2. Wölfle, D., Schmidt, H. and Jungermann, K. (1982).
   Eur.J. Biochem 135,   405 - 412
3. Speth, M. and Schulze, H.-U. (1981). Biochem.
   Biophys. Res. Commun. 99,   134 - 141
4. Suzuki, S., Toyota, T., Suzuki, H. and Goto, Y.(1984).
   Biochem.Biophys. Res. Commun. 118,   40 - 46

Reprints to:

Dr. rer.nat. B. Christ
Institut für Biochemie
Universität Göttingen
Humboldtallee 23

D - 3400   Göttingen

27
Primary Cultures of Rat Hepatocytes as a Model for the Study of Metabolite Dependent Induction of Liponeogenic Enzymes

N.R. KATZ and S. GIFFHORN

Zentrallabor am Universitätsklinikum Freiburg and Institut für Biochemie, Universität Göttingen

Zusammenfassung

Mit Primärkulturen von Rattenhepatocyten steht ein isoliertes Organsystem zur Verfügung, in dem langfristige Regulationseffekte von Metaboliten und von Hormonen unabhängig voneinander untersucht werden können. In diesem Untersuchungsmodell ließ sich eine Glucose-abhängige Steigerung der lipogenen Enzymaktivitäten ATP-Citrat-Lyase, Acetyl-CoA-Carboxylase und Fettsäure-Synthase nachweisen. Hohe Insulinkonzentrationen bewirkten eine zusätzliche Steigerung. Rocket-Immunelektrophorese und Einbau von radioaktivem Methionin zeigten, daß die Erhöhung der Enzymaktivitäten auf eine Zunahme der Enzymmenge und diese wiederum auf eine spezifisch gesteigerte Enzymsynthese zurückzuführen war. Der Verlust des Glucose-Effektes in Gegenwart von Hemmstoffen der Glykolyse deutet darauf hin, daß ein Metabolit der Glucose für die Induktion verantwortlich war.

Introduction

The carbohydrate dependent liponeogenesis is involved in the homeostasis of the blood glucose level. This pathway is regulated by hormone and diet dependent long term regulation of the enzymes involved in fatty acid synthe-

sis: ATP citrate lyase, acetyl-CoA carboxylase and fatty
acid synthase (1). These enzymes are decreased during
starvation and increased during refeeding a carbohydrate
rich diet. However, in the intact animal it is difficult
to discerne whether the carbohydrate dependent enhancement
of liponeogenesis is due to the primary increase of the
blood glucose or to a secondary increase of the insulin
concentration. Isolated liver systems maintained for
several days are necessary to answer this question.

Therefore the effect of glucose on the long term regulation of liponeogenesis was studied in primary cultures of
hepatocytes prepared from adult rats. Enhancement of the
glucose concentration was followed by induction of the
liponeogenic enzymes to about 250 %. Simultaneous addition of high insulin concentrations led to a significant
further increase, while insulin had only a slight effect
in the presence of low glucose concentrations.

Methods

Hepatocytes were isolated from fed male Wistar rats and
cultured in synthetic medium M 199 containing $NaHCO_3$
(18 mM), HEPES (10 mM) and defatted bovine serum albumin
(2 g/l). Low concentrations of glucose (5.5 mM), insulin
(5×10^{-10} M) and dexamethasone (5×10^{-9} M) were present
throughout as basic culture condition. Fetal calf serum
3 % (v/v) was added only for the first 4 h of culture.
Incubation was carried out at 37°C under CO_2 (5 %), O_2
(13 %) and N_2 (82 %); the medium was changed every 24 h.
The induction period was initiated by enhancement of the
glucose or insulin concentration after the medium change
at 24 h. The activities of ATP citrate lyase, fatty acid
synthase, lactate dehydrogenase and 3-hydroxyacyl-CoA
dehydrogenase were tested photometrically in a 100.000 g
supernatant (2); acetyl-CoA carboxylase activity was
determined radiochemically in a 30.000 g supernatant of
cell homogenate (3). Monospecific antibodies were used for
immunoprecipitation and rocket immunoelectrophoresis (4).

The specific enzyme synthesis was determined by incorporation of (^{35}S)-methionine into immunoprecipitable enzymes
and trichloroacetic acid precipitable cytosolic proteins
during the induction period (3).

Results and Conclusion

Under basic culture conditions the liponeogenic enzyme
activities were rapidly decreased to about 50 % within the
first day of culture. After this initial period only a
small further loss of enzyme activities was observed indicating that a new steady state was reached. The effect of
insulin and glucose was studied during this period.
Enhancement of the insulin concentration to 10^{-7}M was
followed by a slight increase of ATP citrate lyase, acetyl-
CoA carboxylase and fatty acid synthase activities (Fig.1).
Enhancement of the glucose concentration to 20 mM resulted
in a more pronounced increase of the enzyme activities.The
most prominent enhancement of the liponeogenic capacity
was observed in the presence of high insulin and high
glucose concentrations (Fig. 1).

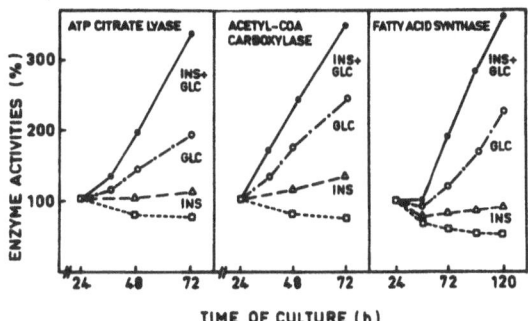

Fig. 1: Glucose- and insulin-dependent enhancement of
liponeogenic enzyme activities. Following an
initial period of 24 h under basic culture conditions glucose was increased to 20 mM and insulin
to 10^{-7}M as indicated. The medium was changed
every 24 h.

The effect of glucose plus insulin appeared to be coopera-
tive rather than additive. Under all conditions the

enhancement of the enzyme activities was about linear for 48 to 96 h. Maximal effects were observed at insulin concentrations around 10^{-7} M and at glucose levels between 20 and 25 mM.

The specifity of this long term regulation was demonstrated by observation that the levels of the non-inducible enzyme lactate dehydrogenase and of the ß-oxidative enzyme 3-hydroxyacyl-CoA dehydrogenase were not affected by the presence of high glucose or insulin concentrations (Tab. 1).

Immunological quantitation of the three liponeogenic enzymes by rocket immunoelectrophoresis demonstrated that the increase of enzyme activities was paralleled by an enhancement of the enzyme protein as shown for ATP citrate lyase (Fig. 2). The specific incorporation of (^{35}S)-methionine into liponeogenic enzymes was significantly increased in the presence of high glucose and high glucose plus high insulin concentrations, while the enzyme degradation remained essentially unchanged. These results indicate that the enhancement of liponeogenic enzyme activities was due to induction rather than to allosteric activation or interconversion.

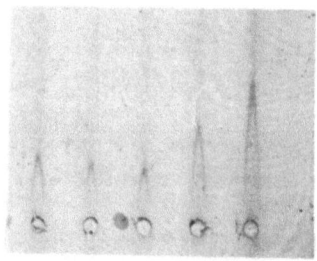

1 2 3 4 5

Fig. 2: Rocket immunoelectrophoresis of ATP citrate lyase
Hepatocyte cultures were tested at 24 h (1) as
well as after a further 24 h period in the presence of: 10^{-7} M insulin (2), basic conditions (3),
20 mM glucose (4) and 10^{-7} M insulin plus 20 mM
glucose (5).

Tab. 1: Specifity of the induction of liponeogenic enzymes.
Enzyme activities were determined after incubation for 48 h
in the presence of 20 mM glucose and 10^{-7} M insulin or under basic conditions

Relative Enzyme Activities %

	ATP Citrate Lyase	Acetyl-CoA Carboxylase	Fatty Acid Synthase	Lactate Dehydrogenase	Hydroxyacyl-CoA Dehydrogenase
Basic Conditions	100	100	100	100	100
Insulin	148	178	139	107	85
Glucose	251	219	208	103	80
Insulin + Glucose	439	455	320	115	89

However, the strong increase of the glucose dependent
induction by high insulin concentrations suggests that
the enhancement was due to a metabolite of glucose rather
than to glucose itself. This view is supported by experiments using 2-deoxyglucose to inhibit the glycolytic
degradation (Tab. 2).

Tab. 2: Inhibition of the glucose dependent induction by
2-deoxyglucose. Enzyme activities were determined after incubation for 24 h in the presence
of 20 mM glucose and/or 50 mM 2-deoxyglucose.
x̄ ± SEM. Significant differences to basic conditions: * p ◄ 0.001

	ATP Citrate Lyase	Acetyl-CoA Carboxylase
	Enzyme Activities U/g DNA	
Basic condition	171 ± 6	79 ± 7
Glucose	$320 \pm 13*$	$164 \pm 8*$
Glucose + Deoxyglucose	179 ± 5	68 ± 16
Deoxyglucose	153 ± 6	63 ± 10

The glucose as well as the glucose plus insulin dependent
induction of ATP citrate lyase and acetyl-CoA carboxylase
was prevented by the simultaneous presence of 50 mM
deoxyglucose, although the glucose concentration in the
culture was even higher than in the absence of deoxyglucose. Further studies will be necessary to characterize
this metabolite which may be responsible for the coordi-
nate induction of liponeogenic enzymes.
The present investigation demonstrates, that primary
cultures of hepatocytes from adult rats are an excellent
tool for the study of long term regulation in liver
parenchyma under exactly defined conditions.

Acknowledgement

The study was supported by the Deutsche Forschungsgemeinschaft.

References

(1) Volpe, J.J. and Vagelos, P.R. (1976). Physiol. Rev.
    56, 338 - 417

(2) Katz, N.R. and Giffhorn, S. (1983). Biochem.J.212,
    65 - 71

(3) Giffhorn, S. and Katz, N.R. (1984). Biochem. J. 221,
    343 - 350

(4) Merrill, M., Hartley, T.F. and Claman, N.W. (1967).
    J. Lab. Clin. Med. 69, 151 - 159

Reprints to:

Dr. N. Katz

Zentrallabor am Klinikum

Universität Freiburg

Hugstetter Str. 55

D - 7800 Freiburg

28

Increase in the Anti-infectious Capacities of Kupffer Cells by *In Vitro* Treatment with Endotoxin*

A. KIRN, F. KELLER, A.M. STEFFAN, C.A. PEREIRA and F. KOEHREN

Laboratoire de Virologie de la Faculté de Médecine de l'Université Louis Pasteur et Groupe de Recherches de l'INSERM (U 74) sur la Pathogénie des Infections Virales, 3 rue Koeberlé, Strasbourg, France

Zusammenfassung

Die in vitro Behandlung mit Endotoxin erzeugt in Kupfferzellen (Kz) von Ratten und Mäusen eine deutliche Steigerung ihrer antiinfektiösen Eigenschaften. Einerseits er-
scheinen neue Eigenschaften, die in nicht infizierten
Zellen nicht vorhanden sind wie eine direkte Hemmung der
Virusvermehrung, eine Komplement-abhängige Phagozytose
und eine bedeutende Interferonsynthese. Auf der anderen
Seite kommt es zu einer Verstärkung von bereits vorhan-
denen Eigenschaften wie die von Kz bewirkte Virushemmung
in Targetzellen. Durch ihre Position im Sinusoid sind die
Kz im beständigen Kontakt mit dem im portalen Blut ent-
haltenen Endotoxin. Deswegen kann eine in vivo Aktivierung
zustande kommen, die eine wichtige Rolle in den Abwehr-
mechanismen spielt.

Several substances are able to induce macrophage activation thereby leading to an increase in their anti-infectious capacities (1). However, most experiments having
been carried out with peritoneal macrophages, the
behaviour of Kupffer cells (KC) is not known. Since it is
possible now to isolate and cultivate these cells we have
studied the properties of murine KC activated in vitro
with bacterial endotoxin.

202

Material and Methods

Isolation and culture of KC

The method developped by us for isolating KC has already been described (2). In brief, the livers were perfused in situ through the portal vein with collagenase (WORTHINGTON). The sinusoidal cells were then purified by centrifugal elutriation and the KC were cultivated in Eagle's medium supplemented with 10 % calf serum. Twenty-four hour-old cultures were used for all experiments.

Animals

Inbred Wistar rats of 200 g as well as C_3H/Hej, C_3He B/ Fej and A/J mice bred under conventional conditions were used.

Endotoxin (LPS)

E. Coli 0127: B8 (Difco Lab) was employed at a concentration of 200 µg/ml in most experiments.

Viruses

Mouse hepatitis virus 3 (MHV 3) and vaccinia virus were cultivated and titrated on L-929 cells and chicken embryo fibroblasts respectively.

C_3-dependent phagocytosis

Sheep erythrocytes first were treated with IgM and then with C_3-deficient SWR mouse serum before being added to KC cultures. The preparations were examined in a Phillips Scanning Electron Microscope after glutaraldehyde fixation and osmium postfixation.

Measurement of interferon production

The interferon content of the KC culture supernatant was measured at different intervals after endotoxin treatment by a classical virus inhibition test using Sindbis virus and L-929 cells. The results were expressed in international units.

Results

1) Intrinsic antiviral activity

As shown in Figure 1, the multiplication of MHV 3 in KC
from A/J mice reaches a maximum 24 hours after the
infection. However, when the cells have been previously
treated with 200 µg/ml of endotoxin, there is a drastic
inhibition in viral development affecting both the
kinetics of multiplication and the final yield.

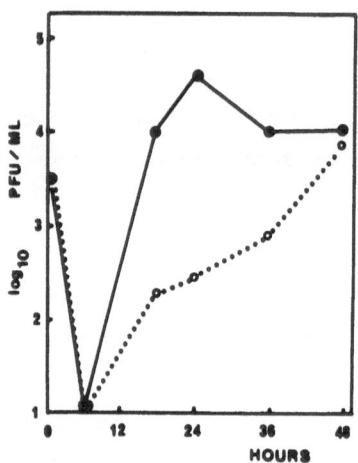

Figure 1: Kinetics of mouse hepatitis virus 3 multiplica-
          tion in cultivated mouse Kupffer cells.
          ○ Control cells
          ● KC treated in vitro with 200 µg/ml of LPS
            12 hours before infection

2) Extrinsic antiviral activity

The multiplication of vaccinia virus in KB cells co-
cultivated with endotoxin-treated KC is drastically
inhibited. This inhibition, which requires close contact
between the target and the effector cells, concerns a
late stage of the virus multiplication cycle (Table 1).
The inhibition in vaccinia virus replication induced by
LPS treatment is much less pronounced when the KC are
isolated from C_3H/Hc endotoxin-resistant mice.

3) C_3 dependent phagocytosis

The presence of C_3 receptors in murine KC allows them to

bind but not to phagocytose C_3-coated erythrocytes. The treatment of the KC with endotoxin renders them capable of internalising the erythrocytes (Fig. 2).

Table 1: Yield of Vaccinia virus in KB cells co-cultivated for 24 hours with endotoxin-treated or untreated kupffer cells (extrinic antiviral activity)

Effector Cells	Effector/Target cell ratio	
	5	25
Control Kupffer cells (1)	$1 \times 10^{5(3)}$	7×10^4
LPS stimulated Kupffer cells	6×10^4	6×10^3

(1) 100 µg/ml LPS treatment for 24 hours
(2) KB cells were infected with 5 plaque forming units of vaccinia virus per cell
(3) The viral titer is expressed in plaque forming units/ml.

4) The treatment of mouse or rat KC with endotoxin induces the synthesis of an antiviral substance displaying the main properties of interferon; i.e., the substance is species-specific, shows no virus specificity and the antiviral effect it induces in target cells requires protein synthesis.

Discussion

The in vitro treatment of KC with endotoxin leads to a significant increase in their antiviral capacities mainly characterized by the appearance in activated cells of properties not present in non activated ones. This is the case for intrinsic antiviral activity, C_3-dependent phagocytosis and interferon synthesis. It is difficult to evaluate the relevance of these activities with respect to the anti-infectious resistance of the host. The intrinsic inhibition in viral multiplication seems to play a role in the resistance of A/J mice to MHV 3, as we have shown previously (3). The extrinsic inhibition in viral multi-

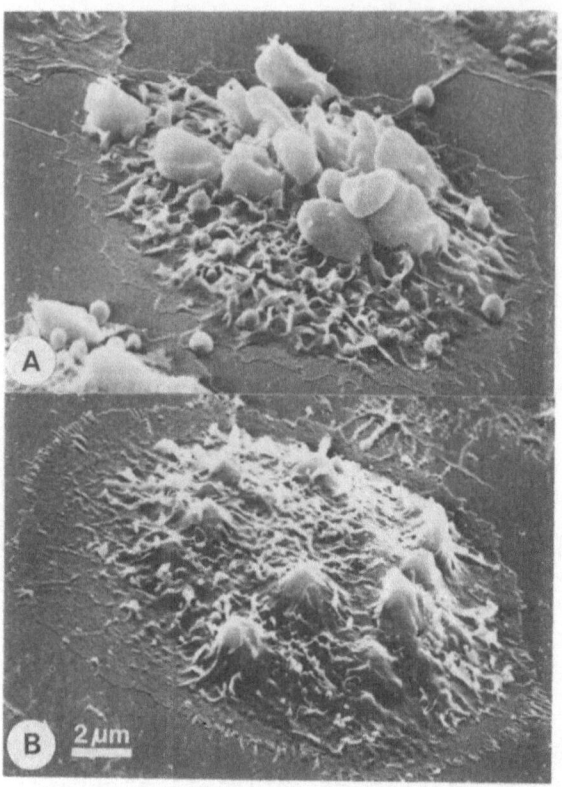

Figure 2: C_3 dependent phagocytosis in cultivated mouse
          Kupffer cells.

    A) Control KC: the C_3 coated erythrocytes are
       bound to the KC plasma membrane but are not
       internalised.
    B) KC treated in vitro with LPS: the C_3 coated
       erythrocytes have been taken up by the cell
       which appears to be distorted by the
       ingested material.

plication may certainly be important in the case of viral
particle dissemination in the blood through infected cells.
This activity is not dependent on interferon since it is
not species-specific and calls for direct contact between
the KC and the target cell. The ability of endotoxin-
activated KC to induce C_3-dependent phagocytosis may also
be a crucial weapon in non-specific immunity as well as in
the resistance to immune complex-mediated diseases (4).
Endotoxin-induced interferon synthesis in KC appears to

be of particular importance; the interferon may diffuse into the space of Disse and reach the parenchymal cells where it possibly produces an antiviral state (5).

The main questions which have to be answered are whether such an activation of KC with endotoxin occurs in vivo and what may be its significance in the anti-infectious resistance of the host in which these cells play a major role (6). Given their strategic position within the liver sinusoid, the KC are in permanent contact with the endo-toxin contained in the portal blood. It may thus be speculated that, the different anti-infectious capacities shown by the KC in vitro are likewise expressed in vivo in the organism when the KC are in an activated state.

References

1. North, R.J. (1978). The concept of activated macro-phages. J. Immunol. 121, 806 - 809

2. Kirn, A., Bingen,A., Steffan,A.M., Wild, M.T., Keller, F. and Cinqualbre, J. (1982). Endotocytic capacities of Kupffer cells isolated from the human adult liver. Hepatology 2, 816 - 822

3. Pereira, C.A., Steffan,A.M. and Kirn, A.(1984). Inter-action between Mouse Hepatitis Viruses and primary cultures of Kupffer and endothelial liver cells from resistant and susceptible inbred mouse strains. J. Gen. Virol. 65, 1617 - 1620

4. Nishi, T., Bhan, A.K., Collins,A. and McCluskey, R.T. (1981). Effect of circulating immune complexes on Fc and C_3 receptors of Kupffer cells in vivo. Lab. Invest. 44, 442 - 448

5. Kirn,A., Koehren, F. and Steffan, A.M. (1982). Inter-feron synthesis in primary culture of Kupffer and endothelial cells. Hepatology 2, 670

6. Kirn, A., Gut, J.P., Gendrault, J.L. (1982). Interaction of viruses with sinusoidal cells. In Progress
   in Liver Diseases, Vol. VIII (H. Popper & F.Schaffner
   eds.) p.377 - 392, Grüne & Stratton New York.

Reprints to:

Professor Dr.A. Kirn
Laboratoire de Virologie de la Faculté de Médecine
de l' Université Louis Pasteur et Groupe de Recherches
de l'INSERM (U74) sur la Pathogénie des Infections
Virales,
3 rue Koeberlé
Strasbourg, France

29

The Role of Kupffer Cells, Endothelial Cells, and Hepatocytes in Uridine Catabolism of Rat Liver

H.-G. LESER, A. HOLSTEGE, J. PAUSCH and W. GEROK

Medizinische Universitätsklinik Greiburg, F.R.G.

Zusammenfassung

Die Funktion von Kupfferzellen (KC), Endothelzellen (EC) und Hepatozyten (HC) beim Uridinkatabolismus der Rattenleber wurde anhand der verschiedenen mittels Zentrifugalelutriation getrennten Leberzellpopulationen untersucht. Die Ergebnisse zeigen eine rasche und effektive Phosphorolyse von Uridin zu Uracil durch KC, während EC und HC in dieser Hinsicht wesentlich weniger aktiv sind. Dagegen ließ sich ein vollständiger Abbau des Uridin zu CO_2, ß-Alanin und Ammoniak nur für HC nachweisen. Diese Befunde sind vereinbar mit einer Kooperation von Leberzellen, wobei vornehmlich KC Blutplasmauridin in Uracil überführen, das dann erst durch HC vollständig abgebaut werden kann.

In rat liver a single pass exchange of uridine has been detected leading to an almost complete removal of the nucleoside from the portal vein blood while excreting constant amounts into hepatic vein blood (1). On this background we wanted to study the role of the different liver cell subpopulations in uridine catabolism.
After collagenase perfusion of rat liver in situ KC, EC, and HC were separated by centrifugal elutriation, according to a slightly modified procedure originally descri-

bed by KIRN et al. (2). Purity of the resulting cell
populations was 90 % for KC and EC and 80 % for HC as controlled by peroxidase staining and latex phagocytosis.
For studying pyrimidine catabolism 1 x 10^6 cells of each
subpopulation were incubated up to 120 min in serum-free
medium (RPMI 1640) after addition of $(2-^{14}C)$ uridine or
$(2-^{14}C)$ uracil. Radioactive uracil and uridine were
separated by reversed-phase HPLC, the peaks were collected
and counted (3). Release of $^{14}CO_2$ after adding C-2 labeled
uridine indicated a complete degradation of the nucleoside. Radioactive carbon dioxide was trapped in KOH and
counted.
The addition of $(2-^{14}C)$ uridine to KC resulted in a rapid
and quantitative conversion of uridine into uracil (fig.1).
After 15 and 60 min extracellular uracil in KC-cultures
amounted to 51 % and 91 % of total radioactivity in the
medium. In contrast EC and HC were much less active.Only
13 % and 36 % of total radioactivity in EC suspensions

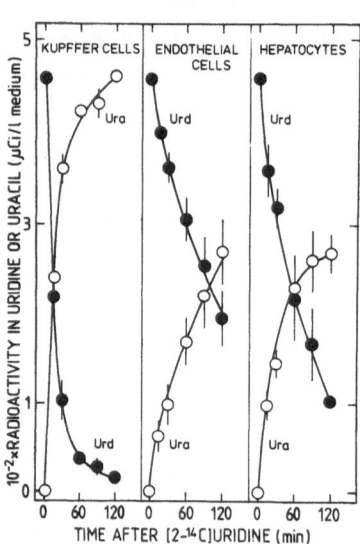

Fig. 1: Conversion of uridine into uracil by KC, EC, and
HC. 1 x 10^6 cells were incubated in the presence
of (2-14C) uridine. After indicated time periods
radioactivity in uridine (closed circles) and
uracil (open circles) was analyzed by reversed-
phase HPLC in the cell-free medium.

was found in uracil after 15 and 60 min, respectively.
When corrected for 20 % contamination by KC, HC only
yielded 11 % and 31 % of total radioactivity in uracil
after 15 and 60 min.

On the other hand uracil consumption by KC, EC, and HC
differed considerably. While KC and EC only consumed a
little amount of uracil from the medium within the first
30 min, HC demonstrated a continuous consumption over the
whole incubation period. Complete degradation of $(2-^{14}C)$
uridine was monitored by radioactive CO_2 release from the
medium. HC showed the ability to completely catabolize
uridine as demonstrated by radioactive CO_2 formation.
In contrast EC and KC did not produce $^{14}CO_2$ due to the
absence of the complete sequence of enzymes involved in
the pathway of uracil breakdown.

In conclusion, our data demonstrate that KC most rapidly
convert uridine into uracil. Uridine phosphorolysis by
EC and HC was much slower. These findings are in line with
histochemical studies, which showed pyrimidine nucleoside
phosphorylase activity to be localized predominantly in
the nuclei of KC and EC (4). Moreover in our own experiments an enzyme activity of uridine phosphorylase could
be demonstrated which was ten-fold higher for KC when
compared to HC. In nonparenchymal cells uracil was the
endproduct of uridine degradation. The further breakdown
of uracil exclusively occured in HC. Therefore our data
suggest metabolic co-operation between different liver
cells in uridine catabolism (fig. 2).

Portal vein blood uridine is converted into uracil mainly
by KC, which are enriched in the periportal area. After
this first step in uridine degradation uracil enters HC,
where it is exclusively catabolized into CO_2, ß-alanine,
and ammonia.

This work was supported by Deutsche Forschungsgemeinschaft, SFB 154, "Klinische und Experimentelle Hepatologie"

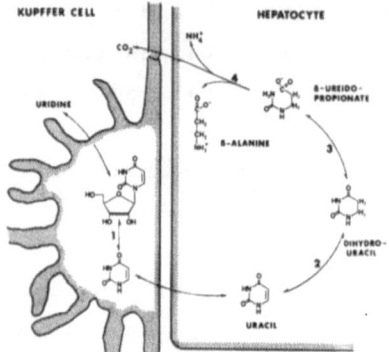

Fig. 2:   Co-operation of KC and HC in the breakdown of
           portal vein blood uridine. According to the
           presented data uridine phosphorolysis occurs
           predominantly in KC, while uracil catabolism
           is restricted to HC.

References

1) Gasser, T., Moyer, J.D. and Handschumacher, R.E.
   (1981). Science 213,   777 - 778
2) Kirn, A., Steffan, A.M., Bingen, A. (1980). J.Reticulo-
   endothel. Soc. 28,   381 - 389
3) Holstege, A., Manglitz, D. and Gerok, W.(1984).
   Eur.J. Biochem. 141,   339 - 344
4) Rubio, R. and Berne, R.M. (1980). Am..J. Physiol.239,
   H 721 - H 730

Reprints to:

Dr. med. H. Leser
Medizinische Universitätsklinik
Hugstetter Str. 55

D- 7800   Freiburg (FRG)

Liver Perfusion

30

Perfusion of the Isolated Rat Liver – Technique and Application in Pharmacology

E. LENG-PESCHLOW and R. BRAATZ

Dr. Madaus & Co., Kölin

Zusammenfassung

Zur besseren Standardisierung der isolierten Rattenleber
wurden eine neue Perfusionsbox und Organkammer entwickelt.
Die Verbesserung der Umgebungsbedingungen erhält den
physiologischen Zustand der Leber über längere Zeit auf-
recht und reduziert die Streuungen zwischen den einzelnen
Versuchen. Zur Ausweitung des pharmakologischen Scree-
nings antihepatotoxischer Substanzen auf Lebern in vitro
wurden 2 Intoxikationen (Phalloidin, CCl_4) an die in
vitro-Bedingungen adaptiert. Man erhält reproduzierbare
Schäden gemessen an der Freisetzung von K^+ und Enzymen
in das Perfusat, an der Verminderung des Galleflusses und
an Veränderungen im Lebergewicht. Das Silymarin-Derivat
Silibinin-dihemisuccinat-Dinatriumsalz antagonisiert
beide Schädigungen.

Introduction

Isolated perfused rat liver in vitro is a method
frequently used to investigate metabolic and kinetic
problems and less for screening of drugs for antihepatotoxic activity. The restricting factor for its application is liver survival depending mainly on the perfusion
conditions. To better standardize the environmental condi-

215

tions we developed a new perfusion and organ chamber. In
addition, we adapted 2 models of liver damage well-known
from in vivo intoxication to our perfusion conditions.

Method

Livers are removed from male Wistar rats (method modified
from (1)) and placed in a swimming position in a Plexiglas chamber filled with a constant volume of circulating
perfusion fluid. The Plexiglas perfusion box is equipped
with temperature and humidity regulation. For handling
inside the box, 4 round windows closed by magnetic locks
are situated in the front pane. In a recirculating system
(modified from (2)) livers are perfused at $37^{\circ}C$ with
300 ml of an O_2-saturated, albumin-containing Tyrode
solution (pH 7,37, flow: 4 ml per g liver per min).
Samples of perfusate and collected bile are taken every
40 min over a 240 min period. Perfusate temperature, pH,
O_2, flow and pressure are continously controlled. Intoxication is induced at the start of the perfusion by adding
phalloidin (500 µg) to the perfusion fluid or by intro-
ducing CCl_4 (1,8 ml) into a gauze-filled glass chamber
mounted into the carbogen stream. As a protective agent,
silibinin-dihemisuccinate-disodium salt (SlHS-Na, 10^{-3}
mmol/l) is added the perfusion fluid at the same time as
the damaging agent.

Results

Perfusion box:
As compared to an older model (3), the more stable conditions in the new perfusion box and the modified arrange-
ment of the liver in the organ chamber result in a retar-
dation of functional losses of the liver due to the in
vitro status and in an improved homogeneity of the
experimental results (Fig. 1).

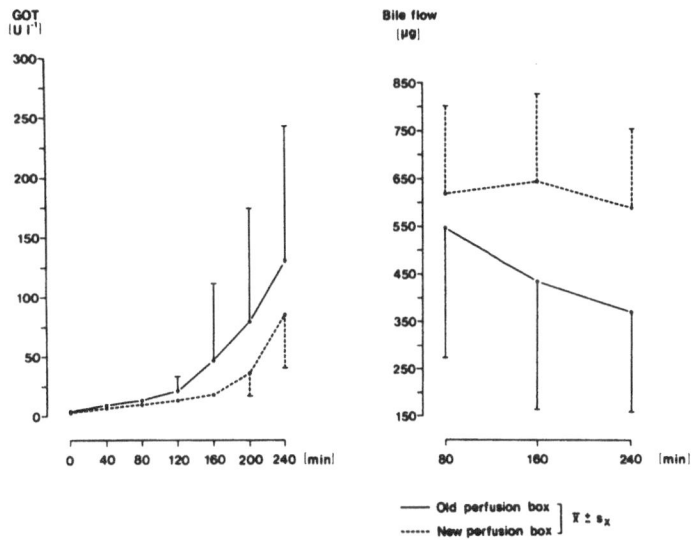

Fig. 1:   Bile flow and release of GOT into the perfusate
          in the new perfusion box as compared to an
          older model.

Phalloidin intoxication:
Whereas non-intoxicated livers maintain their weight
during perfusion, phalloidin intoxication results in an
increase by about 70 %. Loss of potassium into the perfusate is significantly increased already after 40 min.
Bile flow stops completely within 80 min. Liberation of
enzymes into the perfusate, however, is only moderate
during the experimental period as compared to non-intoxicated livers. Treatment with S1HS-Na significantly
improves bile secretion, normalizes K^+-loss, and
decreases the gain in weight to 10 % (Fig. 2).

CCl_4 intoxication:
CCl_4 increases considerably the release of K^+, GPT,
GOT, LDH, GLDH and acid phosphatase into the perfusate.
Bile secretion decreases continously up to 160 min,
thereafter secretion of a fluid similar to the perfusate
is augmented. Lipid peroxidation as measured by
malondialdehyd production is significantly increased.

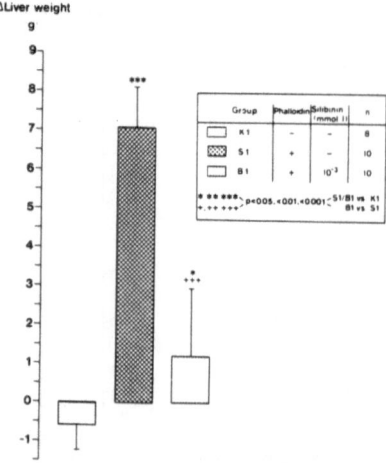

Fig. 2:   Changes in liver weight after 4 h perfusion
          with phalloidin and treatment with
          silibinin-dihemisuccinate-disodium salt.

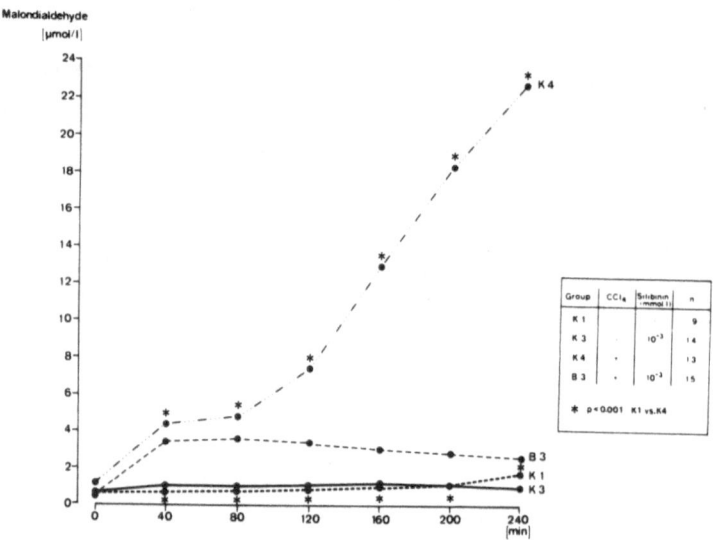

Fig 3:   Lipid peroxidation in CCl_4-intoxicated rat
         livers and treatment with silibinin-
         dihemisuccinate-disodium salt.

Liver weight is not influenced by CCl_4. SlHS-Na reduces
the CCl_4-induced damage clearly: enzyme activities in
the perfusion fluid are lower and K^+ and malondialdehyde
(Fig. 3) concentrations are near normal. The
appearance of perfusatelike bile is delayed.

Discussion

The physiological state of the liver deteriorates
continously during in vitro perfusion dependent mainly
on environmental conditions. Many experiments have to
be done at $37^\circ C$ where decay is rather rapid to better
simulate physiological conditions. Therefore, it is
important to optimize other factors to slow down liver
deteriorization. It could be shown that improvements
of the perfusion box and of the organ chamber
stabilize liver state and reduce variability in
individual results.

Phalloidin and CCl_4 intoxication are well-known methods
for the pharmacological screening of antihepatotoxic
drugs in vivo. They are, however, less known in in vitro-
screening which has the advantage of omitting the inter-
ference of other organs or, simply, of reducing experiments in the conscious animal. The problem of application
of in vivo methods to the isolated liver is mainly that
the action of most damaging agents used in vivo is too
slow to be evident within a few hours.

Phalloidin intoxication in vitro has been mainly established by FRIMMER (4), but it had to be adapted to our
system. CCl_4 intoxication has not been used up to now as
pharmacological screening model in vitro, but our results
show that it is suitable for this purpose.

In addition, it could be shown that antagonization of the
in vitro induced damage is possible by in vitro treatment
with the silymarin-derivative SlHS-Na. It is well known
that uptake of phalloidin into the liver cell requires an

interaction with membrane-receptors and that SlHS-Na competitively inhibits this binding (5). CCl_4-induced damage is due to lipid peroxidation caused by formation of CCl_3-radicals in the liver. The protective effect of SlHS-Na seems to be connected to its ability to scavenge free radicals, thus preventing peroxidation of membrane compounds (6).

References

1) Miller, L.L. (1973). In: Isolated Liver Perfusion and its Applications. J. Bartošek, A. Guaitani, L.L. Miller (Edts.), Raven Press, New York, 39 - 50

2) Schimassek, H. (1963). Biochem. Z. 336, 460-467

3) Ross, B.D. (1972). Perfusion Techniques in Biochemistry, Clarendon Press, Oxford, 135 - 213

4) Frimmer, M., R. Kroker (1975). Arzneim.-Forsch. (Drug Res.) 25, 394 - 396

5) Petzinger, E. et al. (1979). Naunyn-Schmiedeberg's Arch. Pharmacol. 307, 275 - 281

6) Bindoli, A. et al.(1977). Biochem.Pharmacol.26, 2405 - 2409

Reprints to:

Dr. E. Leng-Peschlow

Dr. Madaus & Co.

Abteilung Pharmakologie

D - 5000 Köln 91

31

Drug-derived $^{14}CO_2$ Formation – A Method to Determine the Metabolic Capacity of the Isolated Perfused Rat Liver

Ch. STEFFEN, U. SCHNEIDER and H. SCHULZE

Inst.f.Pharmakologie und Toxicologie, Universität Marburg

Zusammenfassung

Die Bildung von $^{14}CO_2$ durch Demethylierung der (methyl-^{14}C)-markierten Arzneimittel Methacetin, Benzphetamin und Methyldibenzylamin und der intermediär entstehenden C1-Körper Formaldehyd und Formiat in der perfundierten Ratten-leber wurde mit den in vivo gewonnenen Werten verglichen. Für Methacetin betrug die maximale $^{14}CO_2$-Abatmungsrate 1,6 $\pm$ 0,2 µmol/kg·min (n=12). In der perfundierten Leber wurden 1,2 $\pm$ 0,5 µmol/kg·min (n=5) gebildet; für die tertiären Amine und die C1-Körper lag der Wert mit ca. 4 µmol/kg·min deutlich höher. Da für Formiat und Form-aldehyd in vivo sehr viel höhere Werte gemessen wurden, scheint der kapazitätslimitierende Schritt in der perfun-dierten Leber nicht die Demethylierung, sondern die Oxida-tion von Formiat zu sein, die in vivo zu einem großen Teil extrahepatisch stattfinden muß.

Introduction

Drug metabolism in vivo can be measured either as elimina-tion of a drug from the blood or by metabolite formation, such as the exhalation of $^{14}CO_2$ from (methyl-^{14}C)-labelled drugs. This method can be used with a variety of drugs of which aminopyrine (1) is generally used. Parameters that are calculated are the $^{14}CO_2$-exhalation rate (CER) and the $^{14}CO_2$-exhalation half-life (CHL). The latter value is easy to determine, since the exact dose of the administered radio label needs not to be known. In the rat, it cannot be used when the half-life of a drug is shorter than 28 min, the CHL of the common metabolite formate (2). With short-lived drugs, the maximal CER can be measured with saturation doses (3). However, several drugs, such as formaldehyde or centrally active drugs are too toxic to be administered in saturation doses, but can be used in high concentrations in the perfused liver. To evaluate this method, we compared the metabolic $^{14}CO_2$ formation by the perfused rat liver with the values obtained in vivo.

Materials and Methods

Adult male Wistar rats were used for the experiments. The ^{14}C-labelled substrates formate and formaldehyde were supplied by Amersham Buchler, Braunschweig, methacetin was synthesized as described by BRAUN et al. (4), methyl-dibenzylamine from dibenzylamine by the Eschweiler-Clarke reaction and (+)-benzphetamine as described in (5). $^{14}CO_2$-exhalation in vivo was measured essentially as previously described (5), with the modification that 2.5 ml methoxy-ethanolamine in isopropanol (1:1) was used as absorber. The liver was perfused with Krebs-Henseleit buffer (6) supplemented with 0.1 mM l-methionine and 5 mM glucose. When benzphetamine and methyldibenzylamine were used, 10 g/l bovine serum albumin were added. Perfusion was carried out in a recirculating airtight system flushed with $O_2:CO_2$ (95:5), 100 ml/min at $25^{o}C$. The total volume was 100 ml. Collection periods for $^{14}CO_2$ were 10 min. 2.5 ml Omni-Szintisol (Merck, Darmstadt) were added to the absorption vials and $^{14}CO_2$ was measured by liquid scintillation counting with 53 % efficiency. Total metha-cetin in the perfusion medium was quantified by the follo-wing procedure: 0.5 ml perfusate was mixed 1 ml 2 N NaOH

and the absorption at 245 nm was measured after extraction
into 5 ml dichloromethane.

Results and Discussion

The oxidation of formaldehyde and of formate depends on
the concentration of methionine which raises the concentration of S-adenosylmethionine, thus increasing the oxidation of one carbon units to CO_2 by the formyltetrahydro-
folate dehydrogenase reaction (7). Addition of methionine
to perfused rat livers results in an increase of the
formaldehyde oxidation by 50 % (Fig. 1). Therefore the
perfusion medium was routinely supplemented with methionine. However, the maximal CO_2 formation from formate was
only 10 % of the maximal $^{14}CO_2$ exhalation rates observed

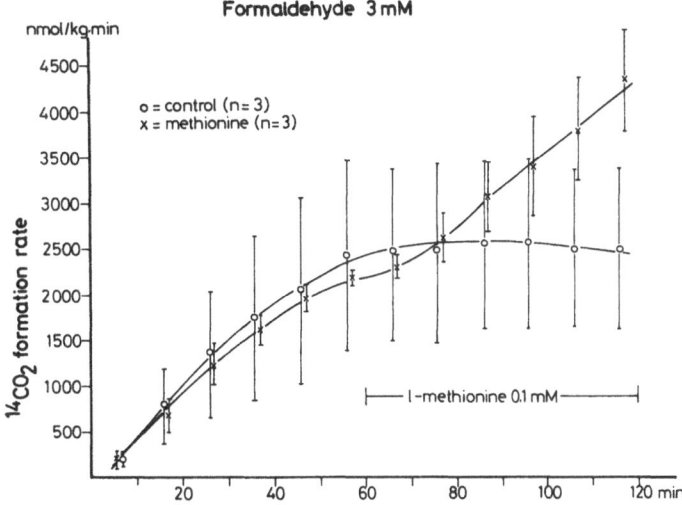

Fig. 1: Effect of methionine on the formation of $^{14}CO_2$
from ^{14}C-formaldehyde by the isolated perfused
rat liver in a recirculating system. The medium
contained no methionine in the control group (x).
In the other group, 0.1 mM L-methionine was
added after 60 min (o), resulting in an
increased $^{14}CO_2$ formation. Data are normalized
to kg body weight and are presented as mean
± s.d. (n=3).

in vivo (Table 1), although part of the administered
formate or formaldehyde is excreted as formate into the
urine (8). Methacetin shows demethylation rates that are
very similar in vivo and in the perfused liver. After a
perfusion period of five min, more than 50 % of the
methacetin are taken up by the liver (Fig. 2). In vivo,
the absorption from the peritoneal cavity must be similarly rapid, since the $^{14}CO_2$ exhalation curve was not different after intraperitoneal and intravenous injection.
The maximal $^{14}CO_2$ formation rate from methacetin (1.2
µmol/kg·min) is much lower than the values observed with
the tertiary amines benzphetamine and methyldibenzylamine
(Fig. 3).

As these amines are very lipophilic, also a short distribution phase can be assumed, leading to high concentrations in the isolated liver. The $^{14}CO_2$ formation rates
from the amines and from the one carbon units in the perfused liver are very similar (Table 1). In vivo,
comparable data cannot be obtained, since high doses of
the amines cause convulsions and death. Both substances
have similar metabolic rates in vitro (5 - 7 nmol form-
aldehyde/nmol cytochrome P-450 min) and are induced by
phenobarbital (9). The maximal tolerated dose for benzphetamine (i.p.) is 30 µmol/kg, whereas methyldibenzylamine
can be given in doses up to 200 µmol/kg (unpublished
results). The latter dose, however, is also not in the
saturation range. Therefore, a direct comparison of the
data in the two models is not possible, but it is very
unlikely that the conformity of the maximal CO_2 formation
rates in the perfused liver is purely accidental. It
seems that the rate limiting step in this model is the
oxidation of formate which in vivo has to take place to
a large extent extrahepatically. The demethylation rates
for the amines in the perfused liver may therefore be
considerably higher than the values given in Table 1.
The measurement of the elimination rates from the perfusion medium is currently under investigation to verify
this hypothesis.

Table 1: Maximal $^{14}CO_2$ formation rates in vivo and in the perfused rat liver

Substrate	$^{14}CO_2$ exhalation ($\mu mol \cdot kg^{-1} \cdot min^{-1}$)	Approx.saturation dose (i.p.) $mmol \cdot kg^{-1}$	$^{14}CO_2$ formation ($\mu mol\, kg^{-1} \cdot min^{-1}$)	concentration (mM)
Methacetin	1.6 ± 0.2 (n=12)	0.1	1.2 ± 0.5 (n=5)	1
Methyldibenzylamine	1.5 ± 0.3 (n=10)	(0.2)*	3.9 ± 0.5 (n=3)	1
Benzphetamine	0.06 ± 0.02(n=27)	(0.01)*	3.2 ± 1.1 (n=3)	1
Formaldehyde	▶ 10	(2)*	4.4 ± 0.5 (n=3)	3
Formate	37.7 ± 14.5(n= 7)	5	4.3 ± 0.9 (n=6)	3

* Administered dose below saturation level

Drug-derived $^{14}CO_2$ in vivo and in the isolated perfused rat liver. The substrates were injected intraperitoneally or added to the perfusion medium (100 ml) to give the concentration indicated in the table. For some substance the toxicity prevented the use of saturation doses.

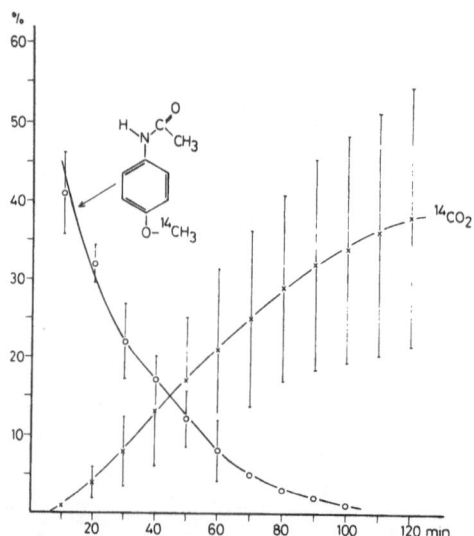

Fig.2: Decrease of total methacetin in the perfusion medium (o) and formation of drug-derived CO_2 by the
isolated perfused rat liver after 3-methylchol-
anthrene induction in a recirculating system (100
ml) supplemented with 0.1 mM L-methionine.After
10 min,60 % of the methacetin are taken up by the
liver. Initial methacetin concentration was 1mM.
Data are expressed as mean ± s.d.(n=3) of the
initial methacetin concentration.

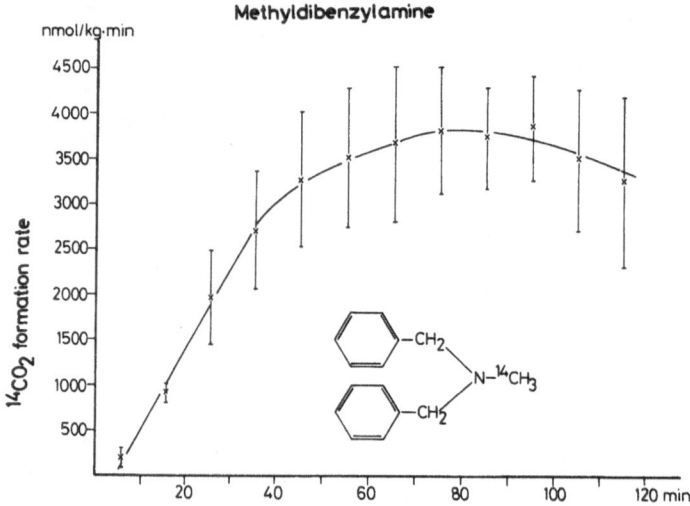

Fig.3: Drug-derived CO_2 formation by the isolated perfused
rat liver in a recirculating system with 1mM
(methyl-^{14}C) methyldibenzylamine,supplemented with
0.1 mM L-methionine.The maximal $^{14}CO_2$ formation
rate is observed after 70min.Data are normalized
to kg body weight and are presented as mean ± s.d.

References

(1) Lauterburg, B.H., Bircher,J. (1976). Expiratory
    measurement of maximal aminopyrine demethylation in
    vivo: effect of phenobarbital, partial hepatectomy,
    portacaval shunt and bile duct ligation in the rat.
    J.pharmacol.Exp.Ther. 196, 501 - 509

(2) Steffen, C., Wittig,M. (1984). Effect of phenobarbital
    and 3-methylcholanthrene on blood kinetics of metha-
    cetin and $^{14}CO_2$ exhalation in rats. Naunyn-Schmiede-
    berg's Arch. Pharmacol. 325, Suppl, R 11

(3) Steffen, C., Friebertshäuser, J.Netter, K.J.
    The use of saturation doses in the $^{14}CO_2$ breath test
    allows measurement of the mixed function oxidase in
    vivo. Biochem.Pharmacol. in press

(4) Braun, R., Dittmar,W., Hübner,G.E., Maurer,H.R.(1984).
    In-vivo Einfluß von Valtrat/Isovaltrat auf Knochen-
    markzellen der Maus und auf die metabolische Aktivität
    der Leber. Planta Med. 1, 1-4

(5) Daniel, W., Friebertshäuser,J., Steffen,C. (1984).
    The effect of imipramine and desipramine on mixed
    function oxidase in rats. Naunyn-Schmiedeberg's Arch.
    Pharmacol. 328, 83 - 86

(6) Krebs, H.A., Henseleit,K. (1932).Untersuchungen über
    die Harnstoffbildung im Tierkörper. Hoppe Seylers
    Z.Physiol.Chem. 210, 33 - 66

(7) Krebs, H.A., Hems,R., Tyler,B. (1976) The regulation
    of folate and methionine metabolism.
    Biochem.J. 158, 341 - 353

(8) Mashford, P.M., Jones,A.R. (1982). Formaldehyde
    metabolism in the rat: a re-appraisal.Xenobiotica 12,
    119 - 124

(9) Sommer, M., Klinger,W. (1980). Age dependent investi-
    gation of different forms of hepatic cytochrome P-450
    in rats: demethylation of benzphetamine and derived
    substrates. Zbl. Pharm. 119, 1038-1040

Reprints to: Dr. C. Steffen, Institut für Pharmakologie und Toxikologie,
Philipps-Universität Marburg, Lahnberge, D - 3550 Marburg.

32
Isolated Liver Perfusion in the Rat – *In Vivo* Model

R. BARTKOWSKI[1], G. HEYDT-ZAPF[2], P.J. HERMANEK[3] and W.J. ZELLER[3]

[1]*Chirurg. Universitätsklinik Heidelberg, Abtl. 2.1.1. Sektion Chirgische Onkologie*
[2]*Fachbereich Chemie der Universität Kaiserslautern, Bereich Lebensmittelchemie und Umwelttoxikologie*
[3]*Deutsches Krebsforschungszentrum Heidelberg, Insitut für Toxikologie und Chemotherapie*

Zusammenfassung

Es wird eine in vivo Methode zur isolierten Leberperfusion bei der Ratte vorgestellt, die die Durchführung von Chemotherapiestudien an transplantablen und chemisch induzierten Lebertumoren ermöglicht. Nach Kanülierung der Arteria hepatica propria und der Vena cava inferior und vollständiger Isolation der Blutversorgung der Leber erfolgt eine Perfusion mit dem Nitroso-Harnstoffderivat Hydroxyethyl-CNU für die Dauer von 15 Minuten. Mit Hilfe einer speziellen Extraktionsmethode waren ca. 60 % der applizierten Gesamtdosis im Perfusat nachweisbar, die systemische toxische Belastung war somit erheblich reduziert.
Nach Wiederherstellung der Blutzirkulation erholten sich die Tiere rasch und überlebten durchschnittlich 12 Wochen.

Introduction

Isolated liver perfusion with cytotoxic drugs has been reported in patients with metastases of colorectal carcinoma and primary hepatoma (1, 2, 3). The advantage of this method is to achieve high drug concentration in the target organ combined with low systemic toxicity. However, the regimens tested are established empirically. A

228

rational base for the selection of drugs and perfusion modalities (hyperthermia, oxygenisation, drug concentration) is missed. An appropriate animal model is desirable to improve clinical results. Experimental liver perfusion studies are carried out mainly in dogs (2, 3, 5), but there are no practicable tumor models in this species. Since we have some well investigated tumor models in the rat, we developed a method for isolated liver perfusion in this animal, which allows chemotherapy studies in transplanted or chemically induced liver tumors.

Methods

We used male Sprague-Dawley-rats weighing 250 - 300 g. Under ether anaesthesia a clean midline laparotomy was performed. Using an operating microscope the hepatoduodenal ligament was split carefully. After isolation of the common hepatic artery, the proper hepatic artery, the gastroduodenal artery and the portal vein a thin polyethylene catheter (Portex PP 10) was introduced in the gastroduodenal artery and placed with its tip in the proper hepatic artery (6).
The common hepatic artery and the portal vein were temporarily clamped with a microclip (Fig. 1).

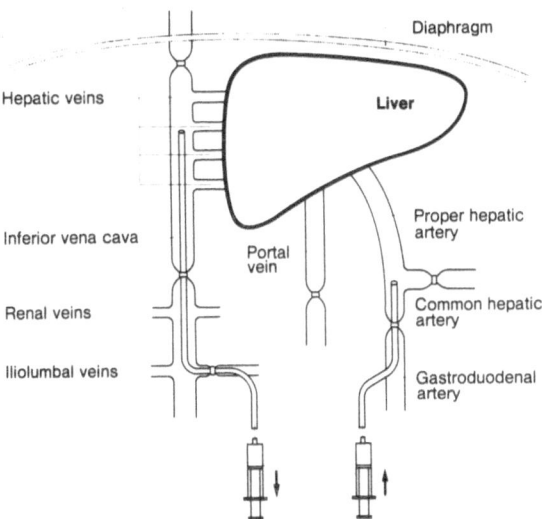

Figure 1: Perfusion flow diagram

Another cannula (Portex PP 30) was inserted in the inferior vena cava via an iliolumbal vein and pushed forward
to the origin of the hepatic veins. To achieve complete
isolation of the liver circulation we temporarily ligated
the inferior vena cava just below the diaphragm and
superior to the renal veins by the aid of silicone
tourniquets, enclosing the catheter, so that its tip was
located between these ligatures (Figure 1).

Additional we temporarily clamped the abdominal aorta
superior to the origin of the superior mesenteric artery
(Fig. 2). This was necessary to reduce the portal hypertension following the ligature of the portal vein in
order to avoid a fatal hemorrhagic intestinal infarction
(7).

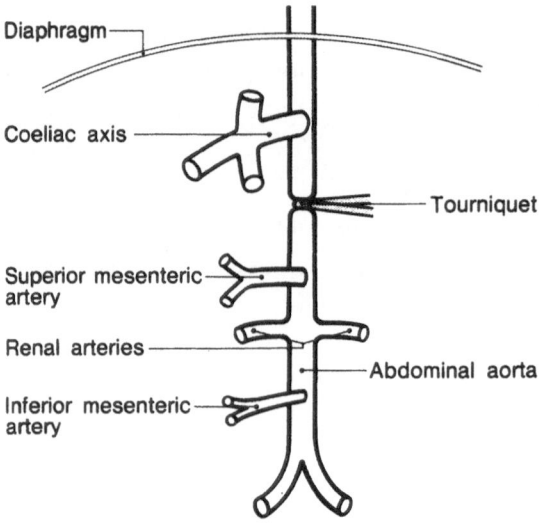

Figure 2: Tourniquet ligature of the abdominal aorta.

The isolated perfusion was carried out for 15 minutes. We
used an open perfusion system without recirculation, the
flow rate was 1.5 ml/min. 5 animals each were perfused
either with Ringers solution or with the water-soluble
nitrosourea derivative Hydroxyethyl - CNU (HECNU)dissolved

in physiological saline (4). The dosage was 10-30 mg/kg
bodyweight. The perfusate was eliminated by the venous
cannula. Fractionated samples of the perfusate were taken
for the determination of the drug levels.

Finally the remaining drug solution was washed out of the
liver with Ringers solution and the blood circulation was
reestablished.Oxygen was delivered for 30 minutes using a
face mask.

Quantitative determination of HECNU:

Individual samples of blood and perfusate (0,4 ml) were
transferred to glas vessels containing citrate buffer pH 5
and acetonitrile (4+1) (v/v). As internal standard
Acetamido - CNU was added.

HECNU and internal standard were extracted after adsorption of the sample solution onto kieselguhr (Extrelut^R)
by on-column extraction with dichloromethane.
Dichloromethane extracts were reduced to dryness under
nitrogen stream and resolved in acetonitrile.

HECNU and internal standard were identified by cochromato-
graphy with the reference compounds after HPLC (UV -
detector) on reversed phase C 18 column and acetonitrile/
water (1+9) (v/v) as solvent system.

The amounts of HECNU in the samples were calculated from
the peak heights by comparison with the reference
compound and were corrected for recovery as indicated by
the internal standard.

Results and discussion

During perfusion with HECNU most of it was eliminated by
the venous cannula. This could be confirmed by HPLC -
determination of the amount of the drug in the perfusate.
About 60 % of the total dose was detected in the perfusate. Immediately after reestablishing the blood circulation there was only a small drug level (about 0.06 mg/ml)
measurable in the venous blood sample. This confirmed the
effectiveness of the liver circulation.

Moreover a considerable amount of HECNU is metabolized or
chemically dissociated due to the biological half-life
period of about 40 minutes.
The animals recovered soon and showed no signs of systemic
toxicity. The median survival time was more than 12 weeks.

The animal model described in this paper is appropriate
for further investigations of the effect of isolated
cytotoxic liver perfusion in the treatment of experimental liver malignancies. It may be useful as a predictive
instrument in the preclinical testing of new therapeutic
regimens.

References

(1) Aigner,K., Walter,H., Tonn,J.C., Krahl,M., Wenzl,A.,
    Merker,G., Schwemmle, K. (1982). Die isolierte Leber-
    perfusion mit 5-FU beim Menschen.Chirurg 53, 571-573

(2) Aigner,K., Walter,H., Tonn,J.C., Krahl,M., Wenzl,A.,
    Merker,G., Schwemmle, K. (1983). First experimental
    and clinical results of isolated liver perfusion with
    cytostatics in metastases from colorectal primary.
    Rec.Res. Canc.Res. 86,   99-102

(3) Ausman,R.K. (1961). Development of a technic for
    isolated perfusion of the liver. NY State J.Med. 61,
    3993 - 3997

(4) Fiebig, H.H., Eisenbrand,G., Zeller,W.J.,Zentgraf,R.
    (1980). Anticancer activity of new nitrosoureas
    against Walker Carcinosarcoma 256 and DMBA-induced
    mammary cancer of the rat. Oncology 37, 177 - 183

(5) Ghussen,F., Nagel,K., Isselhard,W. (1983). Isolated
    liver perfusion in dogs. Rec.Res.Canc.Res.86, 93-89

(6) Leivestad,O., Malt,R.A. (1973). Continuous infusion
    into the hepatic artery and vena cava of the rat.
    Surgery 74, 401 - 404

(7) van der Meer,C., Faber,E.G., Valkenburg,P.W. (1971).
     Experiments of the cause of death in rats after perma-
     nent and temporary occlusion of the portal vein. Proc.
     Konikklijke Nederlandse Akad.van Wetenschappen 74,
     76 - 91

Reprints to :

Dr. med. R. Bartkowski

Chirurg.Univ.Klinik

Abteilung 2.1.1.

Im Neuenheimer Feld 110

D - 6900 Heidelberg

33

Inhibition of Urea and Glutamine Release and of Ammonia Uptake in the Perfused Rat Liver by Stimulation of Sympathetic Hepatic Nerves

Ch. BALLE and K. JUNGERMANN

Institut für Biochemie, Georg-August-Universität, Göttingen

Zusammenfassung

In isoliert perfundierten Rattenlebern bewirkte Elektrostimulation der Lebernerven um Pfortader und Leberarterie
neben der Stimulation der Glucose-Abgabe eine Verminderung
der Harnstoff- und Glutamin-Freisetzung sowie der
Ammoniak-Aufnahme. Durch Infusion von Nitroprussid-
Natrium konnte die durch den Nervenreiz ausgelöste Ernie-
drigung des Perfusionsflusses weitgehend verhindert werden; in gleichem Ausmaß waren dann die Effekte auf den
Stickstoff-Stoffwechsel, nicht aber auf den Glucose-Stoff-
wechsel vermindert. Die nervale Steuerung von Harnstoff-,
Glutamin- und Ammoniak-Stoffwechsel erfolgte also nicht
durch direkte Effekte des Nervenreizes wie bei der
Glucose-Freisetzung, sondern indirekt durch Veränderung
der Hämodynamik.

Introduction

The liver is innervated by sympathetic and parasympathetic
nerves (1, 2). It was shown that in the isolated perfused rat liver activation of the sympathetic nerves
results in an increase of glucose output, a switch from
lactate uptake to output, a decrease of portal flow
combined with a change of the intrahepatic microcircula-

234

tion, a reduction of oxygen uptake and an overflow of
noradrenaline into the hepatic vein (3, 4, 5, 6). The
nerve action was predominantly ∝-adrenergic.
It was the object of the present investigation to
clarify whether the hepatic nerves can regulate besides
carbohydrate also urea glutamine and ammonia metabolism.

Materials and Methods

All chemicals were reagent grade and from commercial
sources. Enzymes were purchased from Boehringer (D-6800
Mannheim), glutaminase and propranolol from Sigma
(D-8028 Taufkirchen), bovine serum albumine from Serva
(D-6900 Heidelberg), noradrenaline was obtained from
Fluka (CH-9470 Buchs), phentolamine from Ciba (D-7867
Wehr) and sodium-nitroprusside from Merck (D-6100 Darmstadt). Male Wistar rats (130 - 200 g) were subjected to
a 12 h daynight rhythm with free access to food (standard
diet 1320 of Altromin, D-4937 Lage). The animals were
anaesthesized by intraperitoneal injection of pentobarbital (60 mg/kg body weight). The techniques of the
in situ liver perfusion with perivascular nerve stimulation (2 ms, 20 V, 20 Hz for 5 min) has been described
(3). Perfusion medium was a Krebs-Henseleit buffer containing 30 % (v/v) bovine erythrocytes, 5 mM glucose, 2 mM
lactate, 0.2 mM pyruvate, 2mM ornithine, 0.2 mM ammonia
chloride (if not indicated otherwise) and 2 % (w/v)
bovine serum albumin. The medium was not recirculated.
All metabolites were measured with standard enzymatic
methods (7).

Results

Perivascular nerve stimulation resulted in a decrease in
urea (-29 %) and glutamine output (-44 %) and in ammonia
uptake (-40 %), reaching a minimum 2 min after the onset
of electrical stimulation. Portal flow was decreased by
28 % reaching the minimal value after 3 min of nerve
stimulation.

In the period after nerve stimulation urea output was
raised by 19 % for about 10 min, while glutamine release
and ammonia uptake remained on their pre-stimulation
levels. Moreover, nerve stimulation led to an increase in
glucose output (+ 300 %) and a switch of lactate uptake
to output (Fig. 1).

Sodium nitroprusside, a drug known to interfere with the
excitation-concentration coupling in vascular smooth
muscle, was infused at a final concentration of about
10 μM starting 2 min before nerve stimulation. Then nerve
stimulation only slightly diminished portal flow and had
no longer any effects on urea, glutamine and ammonia
exchange; the enhancement of glucose release and the
switch of lactate uptake to output, however, remained
unchanged (Fig. 1).

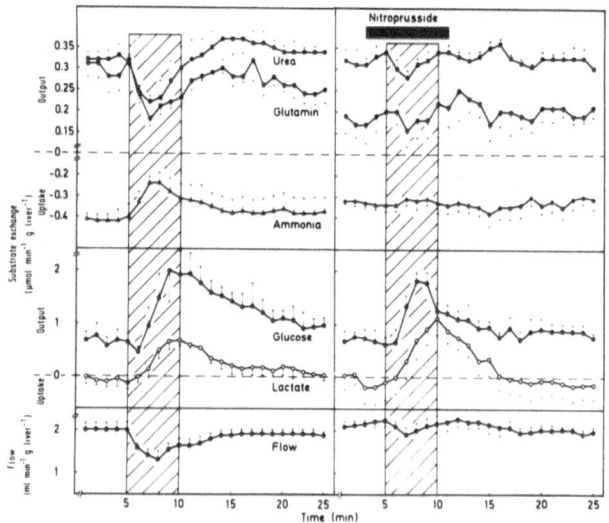

Fig. 1: <u>Regulation of substrate exchange and portal flow</u>
<u>in rat liver perfused in situ by perivascular</u>
<u>nerve stimulation.</u> Sodium nitroprusside (10 uM)
was added for the indicate period. Hatched
columns represent periods of nerve stimulation.
Values are means ± SEM of 3 or 4 experiments.

Table 1: Nervous regulation of the metabolism of nitrogenous compounds and carbohydrates and of portal flow via α-adrenergic receptors in rat liver perfused in situ.

Perivascular nerve bundles were electrically stimulated for 5 min starting 35 min after onset of perfusion. Phentolamine 50 μM or propranolol 20 μM were added, when indicated, at the start of the experiment. The differences in substrate exchange or portal flow is the difference between 0 min and 2 min (urea, glutamine, ammonia), 3 min (portal flow), 4 min (glucose) or 5 min (lactate) after electrical stimulation. Statistics:, Student's t-test: ^{a} p < 0.025 ^{b} p < 0.05. Values are means $\pm$ SEM of 3 experiments each.

	Decrease in			Increase in		Decrease in
	Urea output	glutamine output	ammonia uptake	glucose output	lactate output	flow
	nmol × min^{-1} × g liver^{-1}			μmol × min^{-1} × g liver^{-1}		ml × min^{-1} × g liver^{-1}
Control	90±14	140±12	160±28	1.35±0.51	0.8 ±0.09	0.56±0.01
α-Blocking agent (phentolamine)	20±10^a	30±26^b	40±20^a	0.01±0.09^a	0.22±0.15^a	0.15±0.06^a
β-Blocking agent (propranolol)	140±26	50± 3	160±10	0.42±0.22	0.68±0.05	0.62±0.10

Addition of the ∝-blocking agent phentolamine to the
perfusion medium clearly reduced or abolished all
alterations after nerve stimulation, while the ß-
blocking agent propranolol was effective only to a
minor extent (Tab. 1).

Infusion of noradrenaline could imitate the effect of
nerve stimulation only in part. At 0.1 µM noradrenaline
portal flow and urea output were only slightly decreased,
while glutamine output and ammonia uptake were reduced in
an extent similar to that seen with perivascular nerve
stimulation. 1 µM noradrenaline produced similar effects
as nerve stimulation; the time for reaching peak values
after the stimulus, however, was prolonged by 2 - 3 min,
and the poststimulation increase in urea output was more
pronounced (Fig. 2).

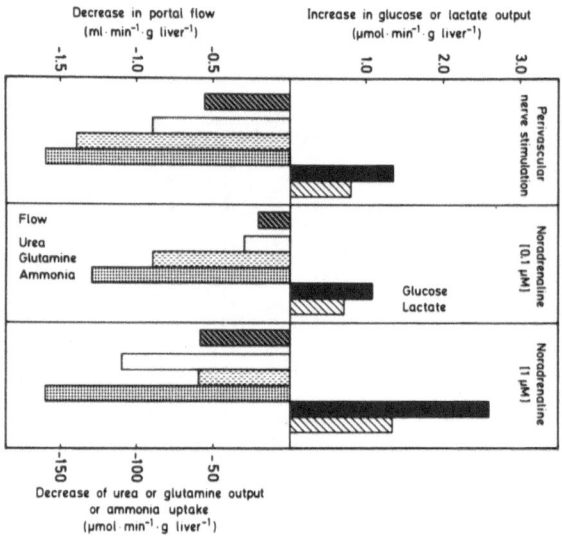

Fig. 2: Comparison of the effects of nerve stimulation
        and noradrenaline infusion on portal flow and
        substrate exchange. Nerve stimulation or nor-
        adrenaline infusion was performed for 5 min (see
        Fig. 1). The alterations in the various para-
        meters are the differences between the basal
        value before and the maximal value after the
        stimuli.

In absence of ammonia in the perfusion medium urea and glutamine release reached only about half the values of control experiments. However, the alterations of substrate exchange upon nerve stimulation remained essentially unchanged (Table 2).

Discussion

Stimulation of α-sympathetic liver nerves resulted in a decrease of urea and glutamine output and of ammonia uptake. All these effects were abolished by preventing the hemodynamic changes after perivascular stimulation. It was therefore concluded that the sympathetic nerves did not influence urea, glutamine and ammonia metabolism via direct interaction with parenchymal cells, but via a redistribution of intrahepatic flow, which reduced the perfused parenchymal mass (6).

The physiological relevance of reduced urea and glutamine output and ammonia uptake after α-adrenergic stimuli is not clear.

Since liver does not only serve as a center of metabolism, but also as a passive and active reservoir of blood (8), it can be assumed that under certain stress conditions supply of the organism with blood is more important than detoxification of ammonia. Reduced formation of urea and glutamine might be the "price" that has to be paid then. In short-term stress situations the reduced capacity (about 30-40 %) of the liver in urea, glutamine and ammonia metabolism may not be of quantitative importance. In long-term stress situations the observed "escape phenomenon" in the decrease of portal flow and metabolism of the nitrogeneous compounds may be a mechanism of protection: The decrease in detoxification capacity can last at the most for a few minutes.

Table 2: Alterations of substrate exchange after perivascular nerve stimulation in livers perfused in situ with an without ammonia.

Perivascular nerve stimulation was performed for 5 min starting 35 min after onset of perfusion. There was no measurable ammonia release in experiments performed without ammonia. With respect to lactate exchange or portal flow there was no difference between perfusions with and without ammonia.
Values are means $\pm$ SEM of 3 experiments each.

Conditions	Output of					
	urea		glutamine		glucose	
	pre[a]	post[b]	pre[a]	post[b]	pre[a]	post[c]
	nmol x min^{-1} x g liver^{-1}				μmol x min^{-1} x g liver^{-1}	
no ammonia	200 $\pm$ 22	90 $\pm$ 14	167 $\pm$ 29	110 $\pm$ 24	0.38 $\pm$ 0.04	1.71 $\pm$ 0.15
+ ammonia	310 $\pm$ 29	220 $\pm$ 15	320 $\pm$ 9	180 $\pm$ 15	0.64 $\pm$ 0.17	1.93 $\pm$ 0.40

[a] pre = 1 min before the onset of stimulation
[b] post = 2 min after the onset of stimulation
[c] post = 6 min after the onset of stimulation

References

(1) Lautt, W.W. (1980). Can.J.Physiol.Pharmacol.58,105-123

(2) Lautt, W.W. (1983). Progr.Neurobio. 21, 323-348

(3) Haartmann,H., Beckh,K. and Jungermann, K. (1982). Eur.J.Biochem. 123, 521 - 526

(4) Hartmann,H., Balks,H.J. and Jungermann,K. (1982). FEBS Lett. 149, 261 - 265

(5) Beckh, H., Hartmann,H., Jungermann,K. and Scholz,R. (1984). Pflügers. Arch. 401, 104 - 106

(6) Ji, S., Beckh,K. and Jungermann,K. (1984). FEBS Lett. 167, 117 - 122

(7) Bergmeyer,H.U. (1974). Methods of Enzymatic Analysis, Academic Press, New York

(8) Richardson,P.D.J. and Withrington, P.G. (1982). Ann. Rev. Physiol. 44, 57 - 69

Acknowledgement

This work was supported by grants from the Deutsche Forschungsgemeinschaft, D-5300 Bonn. We thank Mrs. I. Rother and R. Otto for their excellent technical assistance.

Reprints to:

Dr. med. C. Balle
Institut für Biochemie
Universität Göttingen
Humboldtallee 23

D - 3400 Göttingen

34
Zonation of Carbohydrate Metabolizing Enzymes in Liver of Diabetic Rats

B. WITTIG, H. MIETHKE, A. NATH and K. JUNGERMANN

Institut für Biochemie, Georg-August-Universität Göttingen

Zusammenfassung

Die Aktivität und zonale Verteilung von 4 Schlüssel-
enzymen des Kohlenhydratstoffwechsels wurden in Lebern
alloxan-diabetischer Ratten untersucht: Die Aktivität der
glucogenen Phosphoenolpyruvat-Carboxykinase war auf 320 %
erhöht, wobei der normale zonale Gradient von 3 : 1
(periportal:perivenös), gemessen mit der Mikrodissektions-
technik, auf rund 4:1 gesteigert war. Die Aktivität der
Glucose-6-phosphatase war auf 150 % erhöht, wobei in der
histochemischen Darstellung keine Veränderung des von
periportal nach perivenös abfallenden Gradienten nachweisbar war. Die Aktivität der Pyruvat-Kinase L war auf 75 %
erniedrigt, der zonale Gradient nach Mikrodissektions-
bestimmung von normal 1:1,7 (periportal nach perivenös)
war auf 1:1,4 vermindert. Das Citrat-Zyklus-Enzym
Succinat-Dehydrogenase blieb in der Gesamtaktivität und
der zonalen Verteilung unverändert.

Die Veränderungen zeigen, daß im Insulin-Mangel-Diabetes
die glucogene Kapazität periportal stark gesteigert und
die glykolytische Kapazität perivenös vermindert war. Im
Gegensatz zum Fasten ist im Diabetes die Glucostat-Funk-
tion der Leber nicht aufgehoben, sondern nur stark beeinträchtigt.

242

Introduction

The liver as the glucostat of the organism catalyses gluconeogenesis or glycolysis. In accord with the heterogeneous distribution of the key enzymes gluconeogenesis should be catalysed preferentially by the periportal and glycolysis by the perivenous zone (1). The zonation of enzymes is known to be dynamic, it changes upon longer lasting alterations of the metabolic situation such as during starvation (2-4). The hepatocellular heterogeneity in diabetes is unknown, its investigation was therefore the object of the present study.

Materials and Methods

Rats were made diabetic with alloxan (60 mg/kg body weight). 24 h and 48 h after injection blood glucose, acetoacetate, ß-hydroxybutyrate, liver glycogen, portal and hepatic vein insulin and glucagon were determined with standard procedures (5), and by radioimmunoassay, respectively. Enzyme assays in liver homogenates were carried out as described previously (6). Pyruvate kinase type L was differentiated from type M2 with a specific anti-PK_L-antibody. Microdissection was carried out as described by Lowry and Passonnau (7). Microassays were performed for pyruvate kinase type L (4) and phosphoenolpyruvate carboxykinase (2) in modified form as described.

Results

48 h after alloxan injection blood glucose, acetoacetate and ß-hydroxybutyrate were increased by more than 5-fold and liver glycogen was decreased to about 10 %. All values had reached intermediate levels after 24 h. Portal vein insulin concentrations were reduced to below 10 % of normal, and portal glucagon was increased to almost 200 % after 48 h.

In the diabetic state (48 h) the gluconeogenic enzymes phosphoenolpyruvate carboxykinase and glucose-6-phospha-

tase were increased to about 300 % and 150 %, respectively, and the glycolytic enzymes, pyruvate kinase type L
and glucokinase were decreased to 75 % and 50 %, respectively (Fig. 1). Similar to intermediate levels of substrates (see above) enzyme activities had reached intermediate values 24 h after alloxan treatment. Succinate
dehydrogenase remained unchanged (not shown).

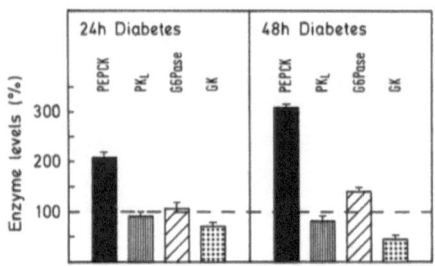

Fig. 1: Specific activities of phosphoenolpyruvate
         carboxykinase (PEPCK), pyruvate kinase L (PK$_L$),
         glucose-6-phosphatase (G-6-Pase) and glucokinase
         (GK) in liver of diabetic rats. Values of control
         rats were set equal to 100 %.
         Columns represent means $\pm$ SD. 6-9 determinations
         were made in samples from at least 3 animals.

The zonal distribution of phosphoenolpyruvate carboxykinase and pyruvate kinase were determined with the
microdissection techniques (Table 1). In the diabetic
state phosphoenolpyruvate carboxykinase was strongly
increased in both the periportal and the perivenous
zone with some predominance in the former area, so that
the gradient in diabetes was enhanced from 3.7 : 1 to
4.4 : 1. In contrast, pyruvate kinase type L was
decreased in both zones with some prevalence in the
perivenous zone so that its periportal to perivenous
gradient was diminished from 1 : 1.7 to 1 : 1.4. The
homogeneous zonal distribution of pyruvate kinase type
M remained unchanged. The histochemical demonstration
of glucose-6-phosphatase and succinate dehydrogenase
revealed, that both enzymes (not shown).

Table 1: Distribution of phosphoenolpyruvate carboxykinase, pyruvate kinase isoenzyme L and M in periportal and perivenous liver tissue of fed control and fed 48 h diabetic rats. Mean values ± SD; numbers of determinations in parentheses; number of animals is given as n; periportal (pp) and perivenous (pv); results were compared by Student's t-test; n.s. = not significant.

	n	periportal (pp)	perivenous (pv)	p	pp/pv
Enzyme activity (μmol $\times$ min^{-1} $\times$ g dry weight^{-1})					
Phosphoenolpyruvate carboxykinase					
Control	4	9.7 ± 3.0 (26)	2.6 ± 0.7 (26)	<0.001	3.73 : 1
Diabetic 48 h	3	24.9 ± 4.1 (22)	5.7 ± 0.3 (22)	<0.001	4.37 : 1
Pyruvate kinase type L					
Control	3	50.4 ± 9.8 (15)	85.7 ± 19.2 (15)	<0.001	1 : 1.70
Diabetic 48 h	3	27.4 ± 2.7 (15)	39.5 ± 3.3 (15)	<0.001	1 : 1.44

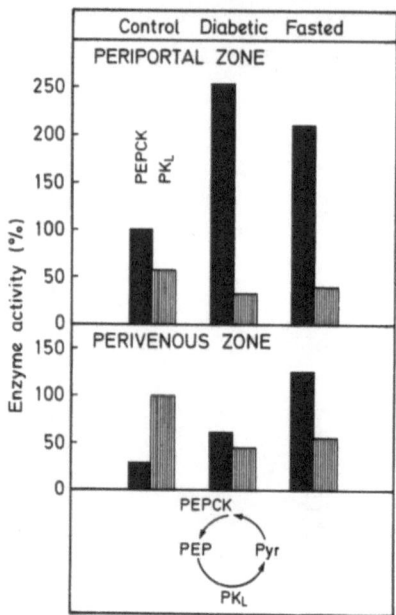

Fig. 2: Distribution pattern in peritoneal and perivenous
liver tissue of phosphoenolpyruvate carboxykinase
and pyruvate kinase type L in fed controls rats,
fed 48 h diabetic and 48 h fasted animals.
Enzyme activities were determined with the microdissection technique. The higher, either portal
or perivenous value of control rats were set
equal to 100 %. The data of fasted rats are from
previous studies (2,4). Columns represent means
of at least 9 determinations from 3 animals.

Discussion

In alloxan-diabetic rats (insulin-deficiency-diabetes
type I) the gluconeogenic capacity of the liver was
increased and the glycolytic capacity decreased. This
alteration was primarily due to a strong increase of
the gluconeogenic potential in the periportal zone with
a simultaneous decrease of the glycolytic potential
in the perivenous area.

In the fasted state the gluconeogenic and glycolytic
capacity of the liver area changed conversely similar
to but more pronounced than in the diabetic state; the
major difference resided in the perivenous zone:
This area was characterized by a "predominance" of

the glycolytic over the gluconeogenic enzymes in
normal animals, by an "equalization" in diabetic
animals and by a "prevalence" of the gluconeogenic
over the glycolytic enzymes in "fasted" animals
(Fig. 2). Apparently, in diabetes - in contrast to
starvation - the glucostat function of the liver and
the concomitant reciprocal zonal predominance of gluco-
genic and glycolytic enzymes is not lost, but only
impaired, since the diabetic, but not the starved animal
continoues to absorb food.

Acknowledgement

This work was supported by grants from the Deutsche
Forschungsgemeinschaft

References

1) Jungermann, K. and Katz, N. (1982). Hepatology 2,
   385 - 395

2) Guder, W.G., Schmidt, U. (1976). Hoppe-Seylers Z.
   Physiol. Chem. 317, 1793 - 1800

3) Andersen, B., Nath, A. and Jungermann, K. (1982).
   Eur. J. Cell. Biol. 28, 47 - 53

4) Zierz, S., Katz, N. and Jungermann, K. (1983).
   Hoppe-Seyler's Z. Physiol. Chem. 364, 1447 - 1453

5) Bergmeyer, H.K. (1974). Methoden der enzymatischen
   Analyse. Verlag Chemie, Weinheim

6) Brinkmann, A., Katz, N., Sasse, D. and Jungermann, K.
   (1978). Hoppe-Seyler's Z. Physiol. Chem. 359,
   1561 - 1571

7) Lowry, O.H. and Pasonneau, J.U. (1972).
   A Flexible System of Enzymatic Analysis,
   Academic Press, New York

Reprints to: Dr.rer.nat. B. Wittig
              Institut für Biochemie
              Universität Göttingen
              Humboldtallee 23   D - 3400 Göttingen

35

Inhibition of Glucagon-stimulated Glucose Release in the Perfused Rat Liver by Stimulation of the Parasympathetic Hepatic Nerves

A. GARDEMANN and K. JUNGERMANN

Institut für Biochemie, Georg-August-Universität Göttingen

Zusammenfassung

In isoliert perfundierten Rattenlebern bewirkte Elektrostimulation der Lebernerven um Pfortader und Leberarterie
bei vollständiger Blockade der sympathischen Nerven eine
deutliche Reduktion der Glucagon-induzierten Steigerung
der Glucose-Abgabe: der Perfusionsfluß und die Lactat-
Aufnahme blieben hingegen unverändert. Insulin bewirkte
ebenfalls eine Verminderung der Glucagon-induzierten
Glucosefreisetzung. Der Nerven-Effekt konnte durch Gabe
von Atropin verhindert werden. Der Antagonismus zwischen
Glucagon und Neurostimulation konnte nur dann beobachtet
werden, wenn der Beginn der Elektrostimulation um mindestens 10 min später lag als der Anfang der Hormongabe.
Die Ergebnisse erlauben den Schluß, daß Stimulation der
parasympathischen Lebernerven ähnlich wie Insulin die
Glucagon-abhängige Glucose-Freisetzung hemmt.

Introduction

Carbohydrate metabolism of the liver is regulated by
hormones and also by the autonomic nervous system (1,2).
In the isolated perfused liver stimulation of the
sympathetic nerves resulted in an increase of glucose output, a switch from lactate uptake to output, a decrease

248

of portal flow combined with a change of the intrahepatic
microcirculation, a reduction of oxygen uptake and an
overflow of noradrenaline into the hepatic vein (3-6).
Preganglionic stimulation of the parasympathetic nerves
produced under anaesthesia in chemically sympathectomized
cats a reduction in hepatic glucose output and an increase
of glycogen synthesis via activation of glycogen synthase
(7). It is not clear whether these effects were caused by
direct action of the hepatic parasympathetic nerves or
mediated via innervation of the endocrine organs, e.g.
pancreas. It was therefore the object of the present study
to investigate in the isolated perfused liver whether the
parasympathetic liver nerves can have direct effects on
carbohydrate metabolism.

Materials and Methods

All chemicals were reagent grade from commercial sources.
Enzymes were purchased from Boehringer (D-6800 Mannheim),
bovine serum albumin from Serva (D-6900 Heidelberg),
phentolamine from Ciba (D-7867 Wehr), propranolol,
neostigmine and atropine from Sigma (D-8028 Taufkirchen).
Male Wistar rats (130-210 g) were subjected to a 12 h day-
night rhythm with free access to food (standard diet 1320
from Altromin, D-4937 Lage). The animals were anaesthesized by intraperitoneal injection of pentobarbital (60 mg/
kg body weight). The technique of the in situ liver perfusion with perivascular nerve stimulation (2 ms, 20 V,
20 Hz for 5 min) has been previously described (3).
Perfusion medium was a Krebs-Henseleit bicarbonate buffer
containing 30 % (v/v) bovine erythrocytes, 10 mM glucose,
2 mM lactate, 0.2 mM pyruvate, 2 mM alanine, 2 mM ornithine, 1 mM glutamine, 0.2 mM NH_4Cl, 50 µM propranolol,
50 µM phentolamine, 1 µM neostigmine and 2 % (v/v) bovine
serum albumine. The medium was equilibrated with 13 %
(v/v) oxygen, 5 % carbon dioxide and 82 % nitrogen; it
was not recirculated. All metabolites were measured with
standard enzymatic methods.

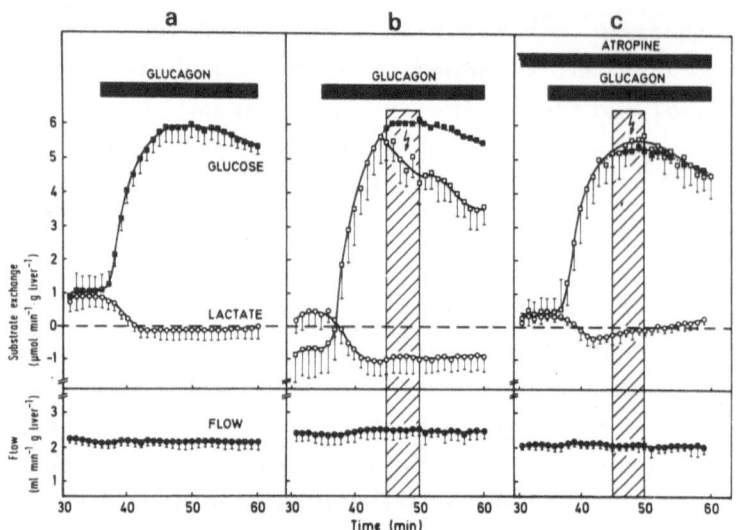

Fig. 1: Inhibition of glucagon induced glucose release
         by stimulation of the parasympathetic liver
         nerves in the perfused rat liver
         (Fig. 1a - c: 1 nM glucagon).

Results

Rat liver was perfused in situ under constant pressure.
The ∝- and ß-blocking agents phentolamine and propranolol
were added to the perfusion medium in order to suppress
sympathetic nerve action. Perivascular nerve stimulation
40 min after the start of perfusion in ∝-, ß-blocked
livers resulted only in a very small reduction of glucose
output; portal flow and lactate output remained completely unaltered (not shown).

Glucagon (1 nM) added after 35 min of perfusion increased
glucose output from 0.5 to 5 µmol x min^{-1} x g liver^{-1}
reaching the maximum 10 min after addition (Fig. 1 a).
Glucose release remained nearly constant for the following 20 min. Moreover, glucagon addition resulted in a
switch of lactate output to uptake and in a slight
increase of portal flow. Perivascular nerve stimulation
10 min after glucagon addition in ∝-, ß-blocked livers a
marked decrease of the glucagon-induced enhancement of

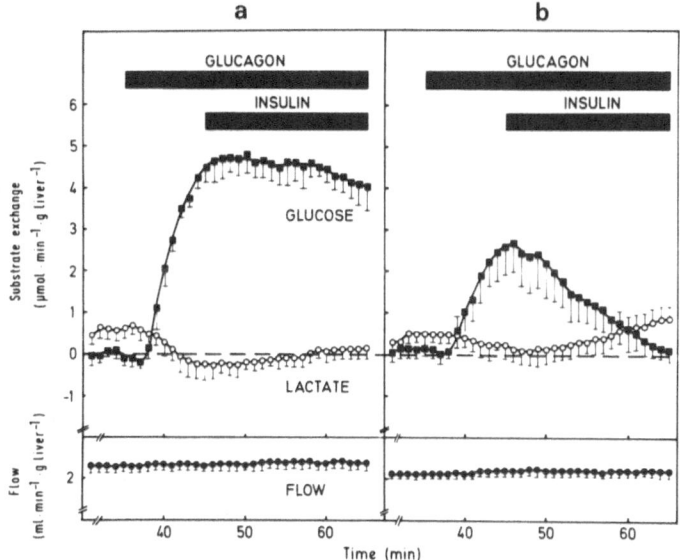

Fig. 2: Inhibition of glucagon induced glucose release
         by insulin in the perfused rat liver.
         (Fig. 2a :   1 nM glucagon, 100 nM insulin;
         Fig. 2 b :   0.4 nM glucagon, 100 nM insulin).

glucose output (Fig. 1 b). Portal flow and lactate uptake
remained constant. Insulin (100 nM) added 10 min after a
lower glucagon dose release, in contrast to nerve stimulation it was not an antogonist with the higher glucagon
dose (1 nM) (Fig. 2). This nerve effect was only repro-
ducibly observable, if neostigmine - an inhibitor of
acetylcholinesterase - was added to the perfusion medium.
The effect was not observed in the presence of 50 µM
atropine (Fig. 1 c).

The antagonism between glucagon and nerve stimulation was
only detectable, when the electrostimulation began at
least 10 min later than glucagon addition (Fig. 3). When
the start of stimulation was retarded for another 5 min,
the effect of vagal nerves was more pronounced.

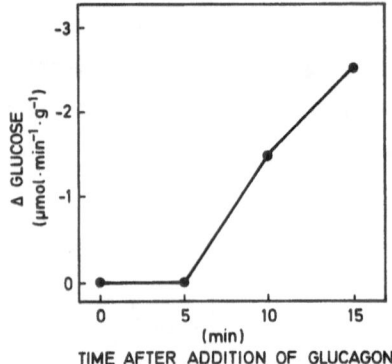

Fig. 3: Time dependence of the antagonism between glucagon and parasympathetic nerve stimulation on glucose release in the perfused rat liver.

Discussion

Stimulation of the liver nerves under α, ß-blockade resulted in a decrease of the glucagon induced enhancement of glucose output. This effects was suppressed by atropine indicating that it was due to parasympathetic nerve action. When the α- and ß-blocking agents phentolamine and propranolol were omitted, the stimulation of hepatic nerves caused a further increase of the glucagon induced enhancement of glucose output (3). Hence the sympathetic nervous system of the liver was clearly predominant over the parasympathetic system, when all hepatic nerves were stimulated. The complete inhibition of the noradrenergic nerves was therefore an indispensable prerequisite for the investigation on the effects of parasympathetic liver nerves on carbohydrate metabolism in the perfused liver.

Insulin very similar to the stimulation of the parasympathetic liver nerves also reduced the glucagon-stimulated glucose release. It can therefore be assumed that insulin, the release of which can also be stimulated by parasympathetic nerve action, and the parasympathetic liver nerves jointly control hepatic glucose metabolism as antagonists of glucagon and the sympathetic liver nerves (8).

It is not clear, why in the perfusion system the parasympathetic nerve action was only detectable after an increase of glucose output caused by glucagon. Nevertheless even in the intact animal the effect of vagal nerve stimulation on liver carbohydrate metabolism has also been demonstrated only as a reduction of glucose output and not as a switch to glucose uptake (7).

References

1) Lautt, W.W. (1980). Can.J.Physiol.Pharmacol.58,105-123

2) Lautt, W.W. (1983). Progress in Neurobiology 21, 323 - 348

3) Hartmann, H., Beckh, K. and Jungermann, K. (1982). Eur. J. Biochem. 123, 521 - 526

4) Beckh, K., Balks, H.-J. and Jungermann, K. (1982). FEBS Letters 149, 261 - 265

5) Beckh, K., Hartmann, H., Jungermann, K. and Scholz, R. (1984). Pflügers Arch. 401, 104 - 106

6) Ji, S., Beckh, K. and Jungermann, K. (1984). FEBS Letters 167, 117 - 122

7) Lautt, W.W., Wong, C. (1978). Can. J. Physiol. Pharmacol. 56, 678 - 682

8) Beckh, K., Hartmann, H. and Jungermann, K. (1982). FEBS Letters 146, 69 - 72

Acknowledgement

This work was supported by grants from the Deutsche Forschungsgemeinschaft, D-5300 Bonn. We thank Mrs. H. Strulik for her excellent technical assistance.

Reprints to: Dr. rer.nat. H. Gardemann
                Institut für Biochemie
                Universität Göttingen
                Humboldtallee 23   D - 3400   Göttingen

36

Inhibition of Ketogenesis by Stimulation of the Hepatic Sympathetic Nerves in the Perfused Rat Liver

U. BEUERS, K. BECKH and K. JUNGERMANN

Institut für Biochemie, Georg-August-Universität Göttingen

Zusammenfassung

In der isoliert perfundierten Leber der Ratte führte Elektrostimulation der Lebernerven um Portalvene und Leberarterie neben einer Erhöhung der Glucose-Abgabe, einer Umschaltung von Lactat-Aufnahme in -Abgabe und einer Flußverminderung zu einer Hemmung der Ketonkörper-freisetzung, sowohl bei der basalen als auch der Oleat-stimulierten Ketogenese. Die verminderte Ketogenese be-ruhte auf einer Hemmung der Acetoacetat- bei konstanter ß-Hydroxybutyrat-Freisetzung. Gabe des α-Blockers Phentolamin hob die nach Neurostimulation beobachteten Effekte vollständig auf. Infusion von Nitroprussid-Natrium verhinderte die durch Nervenreize ausgelöste Ver-minderung des Perfusionsflusses, nicht die der Ketogenese. Infusion von Noradrenalin (0,1 µM) imitierte die Effekte des Nervenreizes auf die untersuchten Stoffwechsel-prozesse bei nur geringer Veränderung der Flußrate. Die Ergebnisse deuten an, daß neben der Glykogenolyse auch die Ketogenese einer direkten Regulation durch das sympathische Nervensystem unterliegt, Veränderungen der Hämodynamik scheinen eine untergeordnete Rolle zu spielen.

Materials and Methods

All chemicals were reagent grade and from commercial
sources. Enzymes were purchased from Boehringer (D-6800
Mannheim), bovine serum albumin and noradrenaline from
Serva (D-6900 Heidelberg), phentolamine from Ciba
(7867 Wehr), nitroprusside-sodium and oleate from Merck
(D-6100 Darmstadt). Male Wistar rats (140 - 190 g) were
kept on a 12 h day-night rhythm (7-19 h) with free access
to food, standard diet of Altromin (D-4937 Lage).
Experiments were performed between 9 h and 12 h. The
animals were anaesthetized by intraperitoneal injection
of pentobarbital (60 mg/kg body weight). The techniques
of the non-recirculating in situ perfusion of the liver
and the perivascular nerve stimulation (20 Hz, 20 V, 2
msec) have been described previously (3). Perfusion
medium was a Krebs-Henseleit-bicarbonate buffer containing 30 % (v/v) bovine erythrocytes, 5 mM glucose, 2 mM
lactate, 0.2 mM pyruvate, 2 % (w/v) bovine serum defatted
albumin + 0.75 mM oleate equilibrated with a gas mixture
of 13 % (v/v) O_2, 5 % (v/v) CO_2 and 82 % (v/v) N_2.
All metabolites were measured with standard enzymatic
methods.

Results

Under basal conditions with 5 mM glucose, 2 mM lactate,
0.2 M pyruvate and 2 % (w/v) defatted bovine serum
albumin the perfused rat liver released acetoacetate and
hydroxybutyrate at a rate of 0.27 and 0.04 μmol x min^{-1}
x g^{-1}, respectively. Electrical stimulation of the nerve
bundles around the hepatic artery and the portal vein
resulted in a decrease of acetoacetate production to 30 %
with essentially no change in hydroxybutyrate release, an
increase of glucose output to 300 %, a switch from lactate
uptake to output and a decrease of perfusion flow (Fig.
1a). With addition of 0.75 mM oleate the production of
acetoacetate was slightly and that of hydroxybutyrate
drastically increased, reaching the rate of acetoacetate

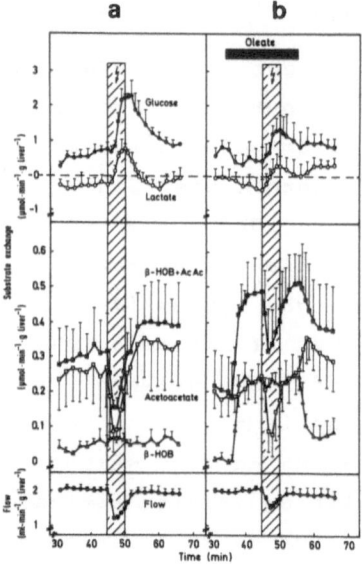

Fig. 1: Regulation of substrate exchange and portal flow
        in rat liver perfused in situ by perivascular
        nerve stimulation under basal conditions or with
        addition of 0.75 mM oleate. Hatched columns
        represent periods of perivascular nerve stimula-
        tion. Values are means ± S.E.M. of 3 and 4
        experiments.

release. Electrical stimulation caused reduction of acetoacetate to 35 % with essentially no alteration in hydroxybutyrate production; the nerve effect on glucose and
lactate output was slightly depressed compared with that
under vasal conditions (Fig. 1b).

Phentolamine (50 μM), an α-blocking agent, abolished the
metabolic and hemodynamic nerve effects (Fig. 2a). Sodium
nitroprusside (10 μM), a vasodilatory agent with no
effect on adrenergic receptors, prevented the changes of
the hemodynamics but not those of ketogenesis after nerve
stimulation (Fig. 2b). Noradrenaline (0.1 μM), an α-
agonist, mimicked the metabolic nerve effects on ketogenesis as well as on glucose and lactate output under
basal conditions and with addition of oleate, but had
little effects on perfusion flow (Fig. 3).

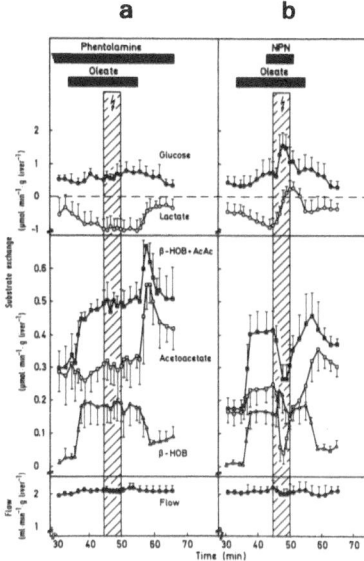

Fig. 2: Regulation of substrate exchange and portal flow
in rat liver perfused in situ by perivascular
nerve stimulation with addition of 0.75 mM oleate
and, where indicated, 50 μM phentolamine or
10 μM nitroprusside-natrium (NPN) respectively.
Hatched columns represent periods of perivascular
nerve stimulation. Values are means ± S.E.M. of
3 and 4 experiments.

The effect of nerve stimulation on ketone body release
showed an "escape phenomenon", in that the rate of ketogenesis, which was maximally depressed after 2-3 min,
began to return to pre-stimulation level during continued
nerve stimulation. The pre-stimulation rate was reached
directly after the period of nerve stimulation.

Discussion

In the present investigation it was shown that stimulation
of the α-adrenergic hepatic nerves resulted in a
decrease of the basal and oleate-stimulated ketone body
release by the isolated perfused rat liver. The effect
was apparently independent of the hemodynamic changes
after nerve stimulation, it can be assumed therefore that
the effect was due to a more direct nerve action on the
parenchymal cells as seen in nerval regulation of

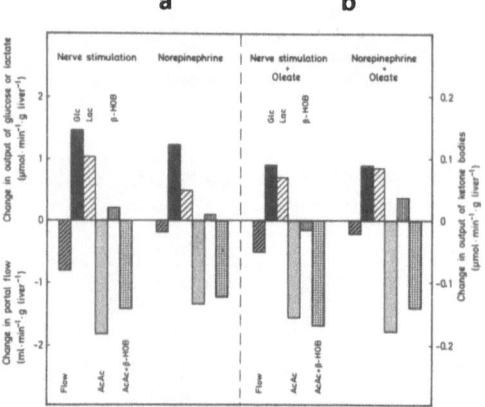

Fig. 3: Comparison of the effects of nerve stimulation
and norepinephrine infusion on portal flow and
substrate exchange. Nerve stimulation or norepinephrine infusion was performed for the period
45-50 min after onset of perfusion. Change in
output of glucose and lactate is the difference
between 45 min and 50 min (stimulation) respectively 51 min (infusion). The change in portal flow
and output of ketone bodies is the difference
between 45 min and 47 min (stimulation) respectively 48 min (infusion). Values are means of 3
experiments.

glycogenolysis (3). The exact mode of action remains to
be clarified.

It is generally accepted that in ketotic states the oxidation of ketone bodies by peripheral organs such as
skeletal muscle predominates and inhibits the oxidation
of glucose (7). The rate of ketolysis seems to be regulated mainly by the plasma concentrations of ketone bodies
offered by the liver to the peripheral organs. During
stronger exercise skeletal muscles require the supply of
glucose both from endogenous and exogenous, i.e. liver
glycogen. The oxidation of glucose clearly predominates
the oxidation of fatty acids or ketone bodies. One could
imagine that one regulatory site for the metabolic switch
to enhanced glucose oxidation in the muscles is the liver
where - besides the activation of glycogenolysis - the
ketogenesis is lowered decreasing the inhibitory

influence of ketone bodies on glycolysis in the skeletal muscles.

References

1) Lautt, W.W. (1980). Can.J.Physiol.Pharmacol 58,105-123

2) Lautt, W.W. (1983). Progr.Neurobiol. 21, 105 - 123

3) Hartmann, H., Beckh, K. and Jungermann, K. (1982). Eur.J. Biochem. 123, 521 - 526

4) Beckh, K., Balks, H.-J. and Jungermann, K. (1982). FEBS Lett 146, 69 - 72

5) Beckh, K., Hartmann, H., Jungermann, K. and Scholz, R. (1984). Pflügers Archiv Eur.J.Physiol.401, 104 - 106

6) Ji, S., Beckh, H., Jungermann, K. (1984). FEBS Lett. 167, 117 - 122

7) Newsholme, E.A. and Start, C. (1973). Regulation in metabolism. Wiley, London. pp 124 - 130, 300 - 323

Acknowledgement

This work was supported by grants from the Deutsche Forschungsgemeinschaft, D-5300 Bonn. We thank Mrs. I. Rother and H.Strulik for their excellent technical assistance.

Reprints to:

Dr. U. Beuers

Institut für Biochemie

Georg-August-Universität Göttingen

Humboldtallee 23

D - 3400   Göttingen

37
Extracorporeal Perfusion with Baboon Liver in Acute Hepatic Failure

C. WALTER, R. HÄRING, J. JAKSCHIK, U. KANIA, E. RENK,
L.C. TUNG, D. WEBER and A. WONDZINSKI

Department of General, Thoracic and Vascular Surgery, Klinikum Steglitz, Berlin

Zusammenfassung

Die akut fulminant verlaufende Leberinsuffizienz hat bei
konservativer Behandlung trotz Fortschritte in der
Intensivmedizin noch immer eine Letalität zwischen 80 und
90 %. Die extracorporale Leberperfusion mit Pavianleber
bei akutem Leberversagen basiert auf der erheblichen
Regenerationsfähigkeit der Leber, d.h. sie kann nur Erfolg
haben, wenn die erkrankte Leber noch eine ausreichende
Regenerationskapazität besitzt. Der temporäre Leberersatz
durchbricht den Circulus vitiosus zwischen Ausfall der
Leberfunktion mit Kumulation toxischer Substanzen und
weiterer Schädigung der Leber sowie anderer Organe. Anhand des wissenschaftlichen Posters wird die Äthiologie
des akuten Leberversagens, die Stadieneinteilung der
hepatitischen Encephalopathie als Überwachungskriterium
sowie die Indikation zur extracorporalen Leberperfusion
aufgezeigt. Das Schema der Leberperfusion sowie das Perfu-
sionssystem werden dargestellt und erläutert. Ergebnisse:
Von 1968 bis 1985 wurden bei 18 Patienten mit 23 Koma-
episoden 30 extracorporale Leberperfusionen durchgeführt.
Bei 3 von 9 Patienten mit akuter Hepatitis war die Perfusion erfolgreich. Abschließend wird die Kasuistik der 3
Langzeitüberlebenden kurz aufgezeigt.

Introduction

In spite of advances in intensive medicine, the mortality
rate of acute fulminant hepatic insufficiency under medical treatment still ranges between 80 to 90 %. Since the
300 to 500 deaths due to hepatic failure in the Federal
Republic of Germany mostly involve young and otherwise
healthy patients, the increasing application of aggressive
management such as dialysis and hemoperfusion appears
justified. With extracorporeal baboon liver perfusion.
ABOUNA, LIE and others were able to achieve an up to 40 %
chance of recovery in cases of hepatic coma.

Extracorporeal hepatic perfusion as a treatment for acute
hepatic failure is based on the considerable regenerative
capacity of the liver.

From Greek mythology we know that Prometheus dared to
bring mortals the gift of fire against the will of the
gods. For punishment, Zeus had him chained to a cliff in
Caucasia and sent an eagle to tear up his liver. In spite
of the dreadful wounds, Prometheus could not die, because
his liver kept on growing back again. PACK et al. were
able to demonstrate that, after partial hepatic resection
or hemihepatectomy, the residual liver is able to
increase by about 50 g daily.

Principle

The basis for temporary liver replacement is the great
functional reservoir and the excellent regenerative
capacity of the liver. Due to the loss of the synthesizing
and secretory functions and especially the detoxifying
function of the liver, hepatic failure results in an
accumulation of toxic substances which in turn have a
damaging effect on the liver and other vital organs. The
aim of extracorporal liver dialysis is to break through
this vicious circle and gain time for the recovery and
regeneration of the damaged liver of the patient (Fig. 1).
Extracorporeal hepatic perfusion can only be successful,

PRINCIPLE OF TEMP. LIVER REPLACEMENT

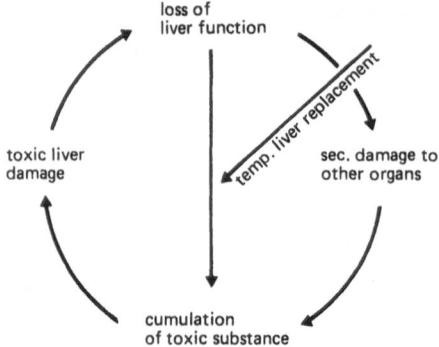

The vicious circle in hepatic coma is broken through by
temporary liver replacement.

Fig. 1

if the diseased liver still possesses an adequate regenerative capacity, i.e., in the acute liver disintegration
not attributable to a chronic liver disease. Chronic
hepatitis and cirrhosis must therefore be ruled out by
laparoscopy.

The ideal organ for liver dialysis is the human liver.
This is out of the question in practice because of donor
problems. We prefer the baboon liver as a donor organ; it
has the following advantages over the pig liver, which
formerly used to be applied:

1. Long-term perfusion possible
2. Slight thrombocyte decrease
3. No humoral antibody formation
4. No "ascites" formation

Indication

The clinical course of an acute hepatic failure is not
predictable; unfortunately, there are not as yet any
reliably parameters for making a prognosis. Above all,
cerebral disorders appear as a primary feature of acute
hepatic insufficiency. We make our diagnosis according to
the stages of hepatic coma determined on the basis of the

classification of hepatic encephalopathy according to LÜCKING.

Already in Stage II, a close contact should be established between patient, hepatologist and perfusion team. Liver dialysis, which requires a great deal of personnel and involves complications, is prepared in Stage III and initiated in Stage IV. If there is a continuous increase in Prothrombin time, the perfusion should already be initiated in Stage III. There is a contraindication in cases of chronic liver damage and a relative one in the presence of concomitant renal failure.

Technique of extracorporeal hepatic function

The superficial femoral artery is cannulated; the blood flows into a reservoir, from which the animal liver is perfused with gravity (15 to 25 cm H_2O). The reflux, accomplished by a pump, takes place via the inferior vena cavy into the great saphenous vein of the patient. The coagulation time is kept at .15 to 20 minutes through heparin administration. The optimal flow volume of 1 ml per g liver weight per minute is kept constant by altering the portal inflow (Fig. 2, 3). To maintain optimal func-tion of the animal liver, systemic blood pressure must be kept constant, high-percent glucose solutions administered and potassium substituted under continuous monitoring.

DIAGRAM OF HEPATIC PERFUSION

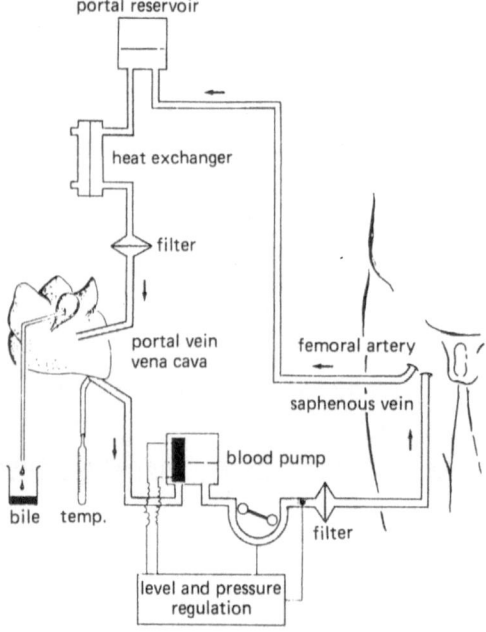

Fig. 2

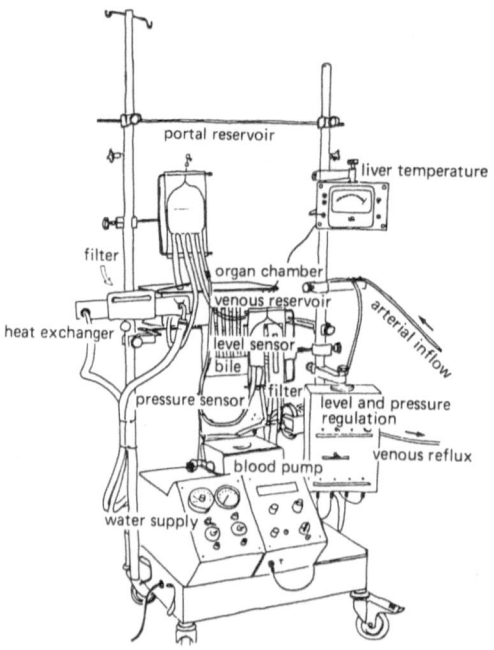

Fig. 3

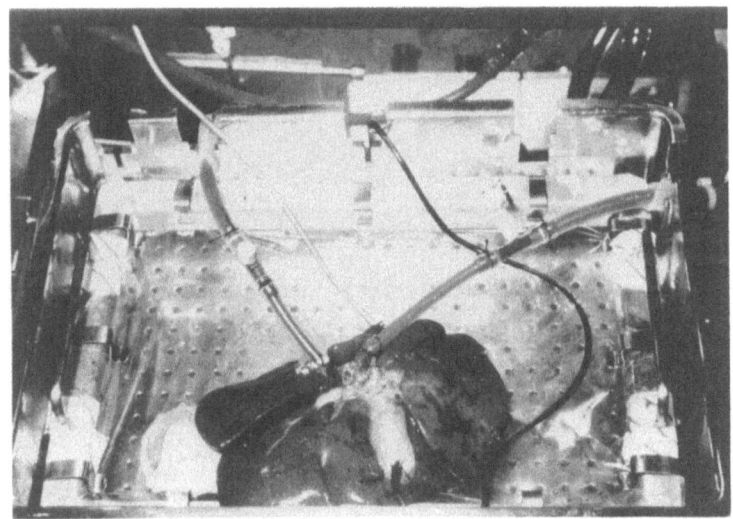

Fig. 4

Fig. 4 shows a baboon liver connected to a perfusion
system in a patient. The liver is uniformly supplied with
blood; oxygen consumption as a manifestation of active
metabolism can be recognized by the difference in color
between the portal vein and the inferior vena cava.

The perfusion is terminated when

1. the patient wakes up,
2. strong bleeding occurs in spite of administration of
   prothrombin complex and fresh blood,
3. the condition of the donor liver deteriorates.

Case report

This 24-year-old patient was transferred to us in hepatic
coma IV/V with fulminant hepatitis; extracorporeal
dialysis using 2 baboon livers was initiated on that same
evening. Duration of the perfusion: 16 hours. After
initial improvement, recurrence of coma stage IV; then
perfusion with a 3rd baboon liver. The patient regained
consciousness after 21 hours and was discharged 3 weeks
later. She has since been completely free of complaints
and working in her profession (Fig. 5).

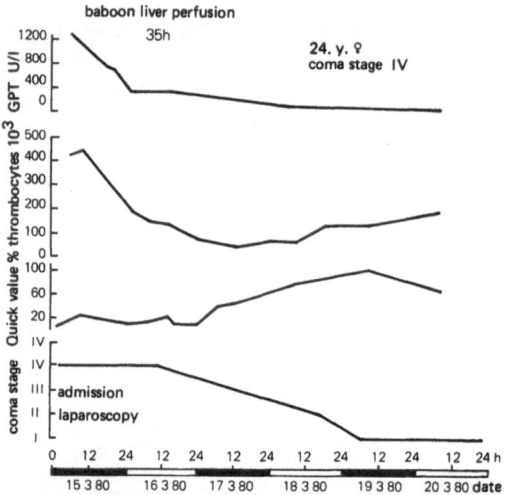

Disease course of a 24-year-old woman with acute hepatic failure, stage IV, in the presence of fulminant hepatitis B.

Cure after 35-hour perfusion with a baboon liver.

Fig. 5

RESULTS:

Results of extracorporeal hepatic perfusion in patients with acute hepatic failure

Pat. Type of liver(s)		Coma episodes after perfusion			
		unchanged	improved	awakened	discharged as cured
pig	13				
calf	1	7	9	6	3
baboon	15				

Causes of acute hepatic failure in 17 patients

	Pat.	Result	
		died	discharged
Exacerbation of a chron. liver disease	7	7	—
Mycetism	1	1	—
Acute hepatitis or liver cell necrosis	9	6	3

Fig. 6

Results

We have conducted a total of 29 hepatic perfusions in 17 patients with 22 coma episodes. The perfusion was success-ful in 3 of 9 patients dialyzed for hepatic failure due to an acute fulminant hepatitis (Fig. 6).

NB: On Nov. 30, 1984, we initiated perfusion with 2 baboon livers for a total of 59 hours in a 33-year-old patient in hepatic coma, stage IV/V. A marked neurological improvement was attained under perfusion; 2 days after the perfusion was terminated, however, the patient unfortunately died as a result of uncontrollable cerebral edema. At autopsy, the liver of the patient was found to be totally necrotic.

References

1. Brunner, G. and Schmidt, F.W., eds. (1981). Artificial liver support. Springer, Berlin-Heidelberg-New York.
2. Häring, R., Waldschmidt,J., Brehme, H., Dressler, S., Eckart, J., Kindler, H., Kotlorz, H., Kühn, H.G., Rena Perez de, R. and Tung, L.C. (1969). Die Behandlung des Leberkomas mit Hilfe der heterologen Leberperfusion Langenbecks Arch.klin.Chirurgie 325, 1123 - 1128
3. Lücking, C.H. Hepatische Enzephalopathie. Klinische und elektroenzephalographische Stadien der subakuten Verlaufsform. In P. Eckert and H. Liehr, eds. (1981). Akutes und chronisches Leberversagen, Schriftenreihe Intensivmedizin Notfallmedizin Anästhesiologie, Georg Thieme, Stuttgart-New York, p. 11 - 24
4. Tung, L.C., Häring, R., Waldschmidt, J. and Weber, D. (1980). Erfahrungen mit der extrakorporalen Leberperfusion bei akutem Leberversagen. Zbl. Chirurgie 105, 1195 - 1205

Reprints to:

Dr. Walter
Klinikum Steglitz
Dept.of General, Thoracic and Vascular Surgery
Hindenburgdamm 30

D - 1000 Berlin 45

38

On Pathophysiology of Preservation Damage in Liver Transplantation

G. OTTO, H. WOLFF, I. UERLINGS, K. GELLERT and W. GÄBEL

Surgical Clinic and Pathological Institute of the Charité Hospital Berlin, G.D.R.

Zusammenfassung

Es erfolgten Lebertransplantationen am Schwein. Für die Flushperfusion kamen kalte Ringerlösung (2°C), warme Ringerlösung (15°C) und ein Blut-Ringer-Gemisch zur Anwendung. Mit Hilfe elektronenmikroskopischer Untersuchungen wurde die Bedeutung der sinusoidalen Schädigung demonstriert. Diese tritt bereits nach initialer Perfusion auf und nimmt nach Wiederdurchblutung des Organs zu. Hypoxie und rasches Abkühlen erwiesen sich als wichtige pathophysiologische Faktoren bei der Schweineleberkonservierung.

Up to now preservation damage of the graft is an important reason for unsuccessful liver transplantation. Out of 29 patients with liver grafting in 6 recipients ischemic graft failure was the obvious reason for death.
With regard to this experience we have performed experimental liver transplantations in pigs. These investigations aimed on elucidating pathophysiological mechanisms responsible for preservation damage. Thereby the phases of preservation with high susceptibility to preservation damage and the influence of ischemia and temperature were of special interest.

Material and Methods

In unselected minipigs weighing 20 - 25 kg liver transplantations were performed. After preparation the donor
organ was flushed via the portal vein with intact
arterial blood supply using 1000 ml of one solution
listed in the table. After hepatectomy and taking the
liver into cold Ringer's solution, flushing was finished
with another 1000 ml. Thereafter the perfusion was
changed to 500 ml of the preservation solution (table)
(4, 5, 6). In group 3 no additional preservation solution
was used.
The livers were stored for 6 hours at 4°C. Before and
after flushing, after preservation, 1 hour and 24 hours
after transplantation biopsies were taken for electron
microscopic examination.

Table: Methods of porcine liver preservation

Group	n	Flushing	Preservation
1	8	Ringer's (2°C)[*]	Collins 2
2	11	Ringer's (2°C)	PPF
3	9	oxygenated porcine blood/ Ringer's sol. (1:1) (2°C)	-
4	6	Ringer's (15°C)	Ringer's (2°C)

[*]Each solution contained 2 500 IU heparin and 250 mg
prednisolone per liter.

Results

The animals in the groups 1 and 2 survived up to 30 hours
only. Survival time averaged 8.3 h in (1), 9.7 h in (2),
30.4 d in (3), and 41.6 d in (4). The difference of the

groups 1 and 2 compared with (3) and (4) was highly
significant (p   0.001).

All but 2 animals in (3) and (4) survived for longer than
4 days.

Before hepatectomy a mild liver damage could be observed
electron microscopically. There were products of hepatocellular destruction within the sinusoidal space
(shedding), a slight swelling of endothelium in some
cases, and a slight vacuolization of the endoplasmic reticulum.

In (1) and (2) the electron microscopic results were very
similar. As early as after flushing the endothelium was
desquamated or it had a high electron density. The
morphologic structures of the Dissè spaces were destroyed
(fig. 1 a). Progression of this damage was only mild
after storage but pronounced 1 hour after preservation.

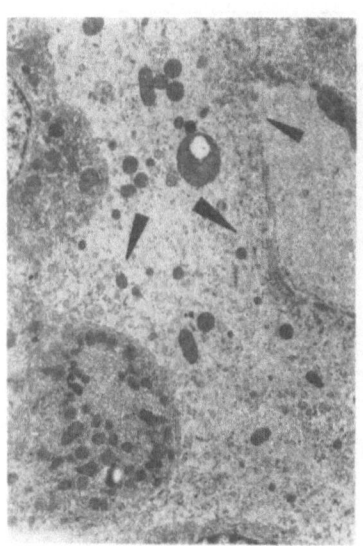 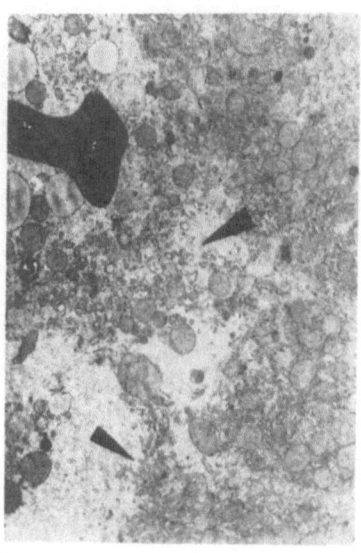

    a   b

Fig. 1: Porcine liver after flushing in group 1 and 2.
        Desquamation of sinusoidal endothelium (arrow) and
        widened Dissè spaces (arrows) (a). 24 h after
        reflow: complete destruction of endothelium
        (arrow), beginning parenchymal cell necroses
        (arrow) (b).

        Magnification 10 000 x

After 24 hours in (1) and (2) the endothelial destruction
was almost complete. Numerous necroses of hepatocytes or
damaged liver parenchymal cells with swollen mitochondrias
and vacuolization occurred (fig. 1 b).

Comparatively the initial sinusoidal damage was low after
blood/ Ringer's preservation (fig. 2 a) and the progression of these morphological alterations was limited. 24
hours after reflow there were only a few endothelial
destructions and widened interhepatocellular spaces.
Parenchymal cell necroses were very rare (fig. 2 b).
Initial and subsequent damage was only slightly more
pronounced in (4) compared to group 3.

Regarding the partially severe alteration of sinusoidal
structures, liver parenchymal cells were comparatively
well preserved. As late as after storage a mild swelling
of mitochondrias and vacuolization of endoplasmic reticulum was visible in all groups. Depending on the damage of
endothelium, these alteration were reversible after reflow.

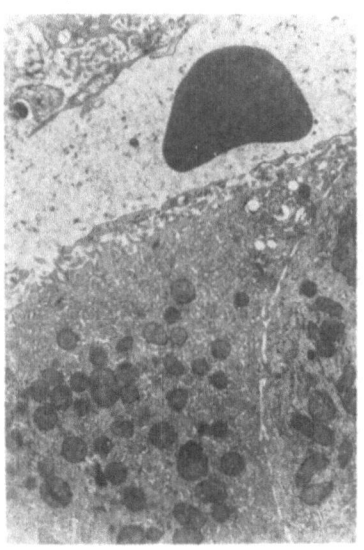 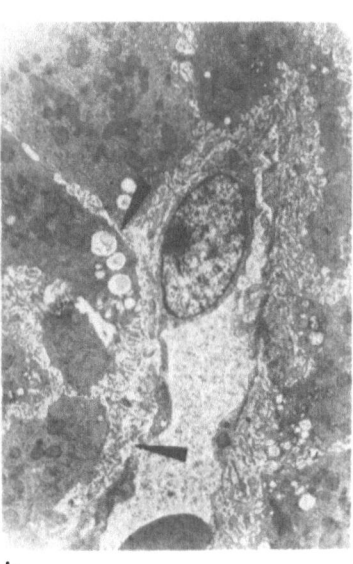

a   b

Fig. 2:   Porcine liver after blood/Ringer's flushing (a).
           24 h after reflow: mild endothelial destruction
           (arrow) and widened interhepatocellular spaces
           (arrow)   (b).

           Magnification 12 000 x

Discussion

Our experiments in (1) and (2) are based on principles
which are used in clinical liver transplantation. These
methods failed in our investigations. This is in contrast
to other authors. Calne preserved porcine livers for up
to 6 hours by PPF (3) and Benichou (1) succeeded in dogs
after preservation for up to 18 hours. In contrast to
these results the survival rate is very low in Bockhorn's
experiments (2).

The sinusoidal damage occurred mainly during flush perfusion and increased after reflow. This initial alteration
could be prevented by administration of oxygen carriers
in the preservation solution of by relatively warm oxygen-
free solution.
The mechanisms of these observations remain hypothetical.
Oxygen carriers may be of importance to prevent an
ischemic damage during the relatively warm phase of preservation. Later on the decreasing temperature limits the
oxygen release from the erythrocyte and the hepatocellular
oxygen demand. Possibly flushing by cold solution acts on
vascular sphincters and inhibits the inflow of arterial
blood into the sinusoidal system. Consequently ischemia
may be an important factor for occurrence of cold damage
too.

After reflow the endothelial destruction increased and
limited hepatic function. Parenchymal cell damage can be
explained as a consequence of disturbances in microcirculation. This was demonstrated 1 hour and especially 24
hours after transplantation. From our investigations we
conclude: (1) Hypoxia and rapid cooling are important
factors in porcine liver preservation. (2) Endothelial
cells are more susceptible to preservation damage than
hepatocytes. (3) Critical phases of preservation are
flushing and reflow. (4) These pathophysiological principles may be of importance in clinical liver preservation
too.

References

1) Benichou,J., Halgrimson, C.G., Weil, R.III, Koep,L.J.,
   Starzl, T.E. (1977). Canine and human liver preservation for 6-8 hours by cold perfusion. Transplantation
   $\underline{24}$,   407 - 411

2) Bockhorn, H. (1981). Die allogene Lebertransplantation.
   I. Morphologische und funktionelle Veränderungen in
   experimentellen Untersuchungen beim Schwein.
   Res.Exp.Med. $\underline{178}$,   79 - 101

3) Calne, R.Y., Dunn, D.C., Herbertson, B.M., Bitter-
   Sauermann, H., Davis, D.R., Smith, D.P., Reitter,F.H.
   (1974). Preservation of the porcine liver.
   Transplant. Proc. $\underline{6}$,   289 - 294

4) Collins, G.M., Bravo-Shugarman, M., Terasaki, P.I.
   (1969). Kidney preservation for transportation. Initial
   perfusion and 30 hours ice storage. Lancet ii,
   1219 - 1222

5) Koristek, V. (1975). Experimental liver transplantation. Acta Fac. Med. Univ. Brunen.

6) Schalm, S.W., Terpstra, J.L., Drayer, B. (1969).
   A simple method for short-term preservation of a liver
   homograft. Transplantation $\underline{8}$,   877

Reprints to:

G. Otto
Surgical Clinic
Charité Hospital
Schumannstr. 20/21

GDR - 1040 Berlin

Index

acute hepatic failure, and
extracorporeal perfusion,
baboon, 260–267
(*see also* perfusion)
alanin aminotransferase, and
cirrhosis, prognosis, 84,
85
albumin, and cirrhosis, prognosis,
84, 85
alcohol consumption, chronic, and
gamma-glutamyltransferase
activity,
alkaline phosphase, activity
and cholestasis,
and chronic alcohol consumption,
aminopyrine, drug-derived
CO_2-exhalation rate,
125–127, 128
ammonia
and chronic active hepatitis,
61, 62
ammonia uptake
and sympathetic hepatic nerve
stimulation, 234–240
and α-blocking agents, 237,
238
and noradrenaline, 238
physiological relevance, 239
and sodium nitroprusside, 236
antihepatotoxic drug screening,
and isolated perfused rat liver,
in vitro, 215–220
antipyrine, drug-derived
CO_2-exhalation rate,
125–127, 128
azathioprin, and chronic active
hepatitis, 68, 70, 71

benzphetamine
metabolism
in vivo, 212, 224, 225

benzphetamine (continued)
metabolism (continued)
isolated perfused rat liver,
222–223, 223, 225
beta-blocker, and oesophageal
variceal bleeding, 100
treatment following
sclerotherapy, 107–111
bile acids
and cholestasis,
and chronic alcohol consumption,
and liver disease, 15, 19–21
after fasting (FBA), 15–21
measurement, 16
after standardised test meal
(PPBA), 15–21
bile duct obstruction,
extrahepatic,
experimental, and liver
energy metabolism
alteration, 3–7
bile salts, and hepatocyte,
hormonal control
alteration, 184–187
biliary atresia, and Tc-99m-IDA-
scintiscanning, diagnostic
value, 36, 37, 38–39,
40–41
biliary secretion
and chronic alcohol consumption,
of enzymes, types,
of gamma-glutamyltransferase,
and chronic alcohol
consumption, 23–30
bilirubin
and cirrhosis, prognosis,
and hepatocyte transplantation,
breath test, 125–130
and isolated perfused rat liver,
metabolic capacity,
221–226